The Child with a Chronic Medical Problem —
Cardiac Disorders, Diabetes, Haemophilia

The Child with a Chronic Medical Problem—Cardiac Disorders, Diabetes, Haemophilia

Doria Pilling

Social, Emotional and Educational Adjustment:
An Annotated Bibliography

NFER

Published by the NFER Publishing Company Ltd

Registered Office: The Mere, Upton Park, Slough, Bucks, SL1 2DQ

Book Division: 2 Jennings Buildings, Thames Avenue,
Windsor, Berks, SL4 1QS

First Published 1973

© *National Children's Bureau 1973*

SBN 85633 027 2

Typesetting and Book Make-Up by
Young Compositors, Burlington Arcade, Old Christchurch Road,
Bournemouth, Hampshire, BH1 2HZ

Printed in Great Britain by
Direct Design (Bournemouth) Ltd., 12 Roumelia Lane, Boscombe,
Bournemouth, Hampshire

Distributed in the USA by Humanities Press Inc.,
450 Park Avenue South, New York, NY 10016 USA

CONTENTS

Acknowledgements

Thanks must first be given to the National Fund for Research into Crippling Diseases whose grant made this review possible.

The Bureau's librarians, Mr. Keith Howes and Mrs. Biddy Cunnell, both by promptly obtaining books and photocopies and by checking any queries that arose over references, facilitated the preparation of this booklet. Mrs. Barbara Forryan provided summaries of several of the French articles included here. A few of the annotations have been taken from Mrs. Rosemary Dinnage's *The Handicapped Child: Research Review*, Vol. II, Longman, 1972.

The Chest and Heart Association, British Diabetic Association and the Haemophilia Society were all kind enough to supply literature which was very useful in the review.

Thanks are also due to Dr. Catherine Peckham, one of the Bureau's senior staff, who has always been ready to discuss any problems that have arisen over the medical aspects of the conditions dealt with in both the present and previous booklets.

Introduction

This booklet is the fourth in a series reviewing research literature on the emotional and social adjustment and educational attainments of physically handicapped children. The present booklet is concerned with three conditions — heart disorders, diabetes and haemophilia — which have very different clinical manifestations and prognoses. They also differ in type and timing of medical treatment. Nevertheless these disorders have often been grouped together under various terms, most commonly as 'chronic illnesses' but also as 'chronic medical problems' or 'special health problems'. Children with these conditions require medical supervision, greater than normal parental care and the disorders are potentially (though often only remotely) life-threatening. The emphasis in modern management of all three conditions is on allowing the child to live a normal life. A number of other disorders might well have been included in the booklet but it was decided to concentrate on the three for which a reasonable amount of research is available. The extensive and complex literature on the role of psychological factors in asthma made a separate consideration of this condition seem preferable. Asthma will be the subject of the next booklet.

This series of booklets — which has already covered orthopaedic handicaps, cerebral palsy and spina bifida — is part of a comprehensive review of research literature (published since 1958) that is being carried out by the National Children's Bureau. The other part consists of three major volumes — on neurological handicaps (R. Dinnage, 1970), sensory and physical handicaps (R. Dinnage, 1972) and mental handicap (D. Pilling, 1973) respectively — which have been published by Longman under the title of *The Handicapped Child: Research Review*, Vol. I, Vol. II and Vol. III.

In the present booklet the research reviewed is summarized in three sections: (1) emotional and social adjustment; (2) family adjustment and (3) educational attainments. In the fourth section, articles and booklets of general interest, including a number on the care and management of children with cardiac

7

conditions, diabetes or haemophilia, are briefly summarized. In each section the summaries are given in date order, starting with the earliest (1958) and continuing to the time of writing (early 1973). They are numbered consecutively throughout, irrespective of sections. At the end of the booklet there is an index in which authors are listed in alphabetical order with dates of works in brackets and reference by entry number.

SECTION I   Emotional and social adjustment

A recent careful study carried out in the Isle of Wight suggests that there is only a slightly higher rate of psychiatric disorder among physically handicapped children without neurological abnormalities than there is among non-handicapped children (Graham and Rutter, 1970). Disabilities of the children studied included heart conditions, diabetes and various types of orthopaedic disorders. There was no evidence of any greater risk of psychiatric disorder for any particular kind of handicap. Nevertheless each of the three disorders with which this review is concerned, cardiac defects, diabetes and haemophilia, has many distinctive features, so that the research literature on rates, type and determinants of psychiatric disorder in each needs to be examined separately.

CARDIAC DISORDERS

There are few studies comparing the emotional adjustment of cardiac and non-handicapped children but, on the whole, available evidence indicates that the extent of problems is not very much greater in the cardiac group. Reed (1959) matched 50 three-to eight-year-old children, who had congenital heart disease, with non-handicapped children and found no significant difference in personal adjustment (clinically assessed) between the two groups. Linde and his associates (1966) found that 198 children with congenital heart disease (average age children with cyanosis, 3·56, without cyanosis, 4·91) differed little in adjustment from their 81 healthy siblings or 40 normal children (assessed by psychologists from the mothers' reports). In a study comparing eight-to 14-year-old children, who had a heart defect which restricted their activity to some extent, with matched non-handicapped children, the cardiac group had higher neurotic scores (Brown Personality Inventory and gave significantly more dependent responses (Despert Fables), but the two groups did not differ significantly in total adjustment (Rorschach)

9

(Neuhaus, 1958).

It is possible that the rate of psychiatric disorder has changed in children with heart defects over the last 18 or so years. Considerable advances have occurred in treatment and many children are now completely cured after surgical operation. One of the major studies on children with congenital heart disease, which was carried out in Finland, (Landtman *et al.*, 1968) found a marked decrease in behaviour problems (as seen by the mother) of children awaiting surgical correction. The incidence of problems dropped from 56 per cent for children seen between 1955-9 to 14 per cent in those investigated between 1965-8. While the earlier figure does suggest a much higher rate of behaviour disorders than would be expected for normal children it is difficult to evaluate in the absence of a control group or a comparable Finnish study of non-handicapped children.

Landtman *et al.* (1968) considered that the main reason for the decrease in behaviour problems in the children was the improvement in mother-child relationships over the same period (the proportion of mothers classified as 'excessively over-protective' dropped from 35 per cent to 13 per cent). The growing confidence in cardiac surgery (at the beginning of the study period only 20 cardiac operations had been performed at the Children's Hospital in Helsinki, while by the end the number had reached almost 1400), communicated to mothers by other parents whose children had already undergone operations, their own physicians and the mass media, probably helped them to achieve better adjustment.

That there is a strong relationship between maternal attitudes and the adjustment of the cardiac child was established not only by Landtman's study but also in that of Linde *et al.* (1966). Findings from both studies also showed that there was little relationship between the severity of the cardiac defect and the child's adjustment. Linde and his associates found that children with cyanotic congenital heart disease (cyanosis is a bluish colour of the lips and nailbeds, due to structural defect of the heart which prevents the blood from getting enough oxygen — such children tended to be more incapacitated physically) were not more dependent or less well-adjusted than the children with congenital heart disease but no cyanosis, although they were inclined to be more anxious.

The possibility of complete or partial cure following operation in children with heart conditions offers a unique opportunity to study the emotional adjustment of the same child both when he is physically handicapped and when he is free from handicap, or, at least, improved. In the Landtman *et al.* study (1968), although 133 of the 200 children in the sample had been considered normal in their behaviour at home before the operation, an improvement in behaviour was still found in 80 of these children one year after the operation. Sixty-seven children had shown emotional or behaviour disorders before the operation (most frequently temper tantrums or crying at night). These disappeared completely one year after the operation in 30 children and diminished in 24 others. Teachers' reports indicated that about three-quarters of the children (out of 104) had improved in general behaviour at school. Landtman *et al.* considered the improvement to be closely associated with the improvement that was also found in mother-child relationships. Linde *et al.* (1970) found statistically significant gains in the general adjustment of children with cyanotic heart disease after operation, although not in acyanotic children. The greater change in the cyanotic children was probably, partly at least, connected with the improvement in maternal attitudes. Previous research had shown that mothers of cyanotic children were more protective, anxious and inclined to pamper than mothers of acyanotic children, although the difference was small compared with the difference in physical incapacity of the children (Linde *et al.*, 1966) and findings also implied that there was a relationship between maternal concern and cyanosis only partially related to the greater incapacity (Linde *et al.*, 1970).

DIABETES

Studies comparing the rate of psychiatric disorder among diabetic and non-handicapped children are also few in the period under review (since 1958). While there are a number of earlier studies, findings from these appear to be conflicting (Swift *et al.*, 1967). In the more recent period the study with the most representative sample of the juvenile diabetic population is that carried out by Sterky (1963). Comparing most of the diabetic school-children in Stockholm in 1960 with non-diabetic controls, matched for sex, age, school-class and father's occupation, he found a similar rate of mental disturbance (assessed by clinical evaluation) in the two groups. Diabetic children who showed signs of mental disturbance, though, had a greater number of symptoms per case than non-diabetic children who were mentally disturbed. The most common symptoms among the diabetics were emotional lability and difficulties with companions.

A study of adolescent diabetics from 58 high schools in Minnesota, US also found no evidence of a higher rate of maladaptive behaviour, as judged from self-descriptions, than among non-diabetic classmates (Collier, 1969a). In contrast, in another study carried out in the United States, a higher proportion of diabetics (50 per cent) than of matched non-diabetics (10 per cent) were given a psychiatric classification other than normal in a joint evaluation by a psychiatrist and a psychologist (Swift *et al.*, 1967). In the same study an independent assessment was made using a battery of psychological tests and the diabetic children were found to have less adequate self-percepts and to show greater anxiety, dependency and constriction. Diabetic subjects were 50 children (mean age 11·66 years) coming from summer camps, clinics and private medical practices in the New Jersey area and, as the authors themselves say, it is difficult to assess how representative these were of the entire juvenile diabetic population.

Evidence for increased anxiety, but not for lessened creative thinking, (both possible measures of constriction) in diabetic children was found in a later study in New Jersey (Del Vecchio, 1971), the diabetic subjects being contacted through the Diabetic Association, hospitals and private physicians. Evidence about the extent of psychiatric disorder amongst diabetic children, then, continues to be conflicting. Until there are further studies, using representative samples, definite conclusions cannot be reached.

It does appear to be established that emotional adjustment can affect the control of diabetes. Studies carried out in the 1940s and 1950s, as well as those of the more recent period (Sterky, 1963; Swift *et al.*, 1967; Birkbeck *et al.*, 1968) all found control to be better in children who were well-adjusted. Swift and his associates found that emotional adjustment was associated with acceptance of the illness and the emotional tone of the home. This suggests that parental adjustment makes an important contribution to the control of diabetes. The influence of emotional factors on diabetic control was also shown in an experiment at a summer camp (Weil and Sussman, 1967), children aged nine or more increasing their excretion of glucose in the urine during a period in which a strong competitive element was introduced into camp activities. Interest in the relationship between emotional and physiological factors in diabetes was considerably greater before the 1960s (Treuting, 1962). A recent series of studies (Baker and Barcai, 1970), though, taking into account new understanding of physiological processes, suggests possible directions for future research.

HAEMOPHILIA

Although several researchers have shown an interest in the emotional aspects of haemophilia, there are no studies comparing the emotional adjustment of haemophiliac children with that of non-handicapped children. The most comprehensive study of children is that of Mattsson and Gross (1966a and b) who observed and carried out interviews with 35 haemophiliac boys (all the haemophiliac children who were attending University Hospitals, Cleveland) over a two-year period. Twenty-seven of the subjects were judged to have made a satisfactory to good adaptation to haemophilia.

A questionnaire survey of all haemophiliac patients who had been referred in the previous decade to the

Department of Haematology, Sheffield Royal Infirmary, found that only 4·5 per cent had received psychiatric treatment at any time (Bronks and Blackburn, 1968). The authors think it unlikely that this proportion is significantly higher than that in the general population. They point out that while a questionnaire survey to patients or their parents may not give a very satisfactory estimate of psychiatric disorder in the sample other findings of the study provided supportive evidence. The haemophiliacs' way of life, for example, differed very little from that of the general population.

One study (Spencer and Behar, 1969) did find a high rate of psychiatric disorder among haemophiliacs. All ten of the adolescents in the sample were found to have various problems of adaptation, including problems of school or vocational achievement, behaviour problems, accident-proneness and sexual or social maladjustment. It is difficult to know, though, how representative the sample was of the haemophiliac population and so no generalizations can be drawn from this study.

An important study (Agle, 1964) investigated the psychiatric disorders that occur in haemophiliacs. Of 16 haemophiliacs, selected by their availability for study when admitted to hospital or attending for a routine appointment with their physicians (no other details of the characteristics of the sample are given), anxiety states and recurrent depressions sufficient to interfere in normal life were found in eight, recurrent risk-taking behaviour in nine and a passive-dependent state in two.

Although Agle's study does not give any indication of how many haemophiliac boys do show passive-dependent or risk-taking behaviour there is considerable evidence that these are characteristics of some haemophiliac children and adolescents. (Alby *et al.*, 1962; Mattsson and Gross, 1966b). The authors of these three studies all suggest that there is a strong relationship between the child's emotional adjustment and parental adjustment. Agle (1964) found that all nine of the risk-taking subjects considered that their mothers had been excessively over-protective. In Mattsson and Gross's (1966b) study there were eight poorly adjusted children, three of whom led restricted, inactive lives, while five showed recurrent risk-taking behaviour. All of these children had over-protective mothers. The other 27 children in Mattson and Gross's sample were all either satisfactorily or well-adjusted and their parents were also well-adjusted.

Findings from a survey of adult haemophiliacs in the United States (Goldy and Katz, 1963; Katz, 1966) suggested that the key to social adjustment in adult life was parental adjustment during the haemophiliac's childhood. Goldy and Katz also concluded that the father plays a crucial role in the haemophiliac's later adjustment. Mothers were to some extent expected to be over-protective and this was accepted by the haemophiliac boy but over-protective fathers were deeply resented. 'Good adjusters' in this survey generally remembered their fathers as permissive or indifferent while 'poor adjusters' remembered both parents as over-protective. Subjects who were forbidden to join in activities with other boys came to think of themselves as being 'different from other children'. In Mattsson and Gross's research, as well, fathers played an important part in families which were well-adjusted. Goldy and Katz (1963; Katz, 1970) stress the dilemma of parents of the haemophiliac who have to make sure that a certain amount of caution is taken over physical activities and yet avoid over-protection. The way in which this dilemma is resolved has a considerable influence on the child's adjustment.

Bleeding in haemophilia is not necessarily due to a fall, bang or cut. Some bleeding episodes appear to occur spontaneously. Several authors have found evidence which indicates that emotional factors may precipitate some of these episodes of spontaneous bleeding (Browne *et al.*, 1960; Alby *et al.*, 1962; Agle, 1964; Mattsson and Gross, 1966b; Garlinghouse and Sharp, 1968), although the physiological mechanism through which this occurs is not clear. It appears to be the anticipation of events, either exciting or stressful, such as holidays, outings or the start of school, that is particularly liable to cause this spontaneous bleeding (Browne *et al.*, 1960; Agle, 1964; Mattsson and Gross, 1966b). There are also reports of changes in behaviour from passive dependence to more aggressive independence occurring, accompanied by an improvement in the clinical state, particularly during adolescence. While it might be expected that the improvement in behaviour would follow an improvement in the clinical state some of the findings suggest that the psychological changes occur first (Agle, 1964), but the evidence is, as yet, inconclusive (Mattsson and Gross, 1966b).

CONCLUSIONS

There is some conflict, then, in evidence about the rate of psychiatric disorder in all three conditions. It is not established for any of them that extent of disorder is very different from that in the general population. Only further, well-controlled research, can allow definite conclusions on this point to be reached. The authors of one study state 'diabetes imposes an additional difficulty upon the child or adolescent in achieving normal life adjustment' (Swift and Seidman, 1964). This sentence is also applicable to the child with a heart condition or haemophilia. Nevertheless it does seem that, despite all the difficulties, a majority of children, at least, manage to cope well.

Perhaps the outstanding finding of many studies of all three conditions is the importance of parental attitudes in the determination of the child's adjustment. While the influence of parent-child relationships on the child's emotional adjustment has been emphasized for many years, the research on cardiac conditions, diabetes and haemophilia stresses this particularly forcibly. Parental adjustment will be discussed in more detail in the next section.

Abstracts

1 NEUHAUS, E.C. (1958)

'A personality study of asthmatic and cardiac children', *Psychosomatic Medicine*, 20, 3, 181—6.

Asthmatic children, children with cardiac defects, normal children and siblings of the chronically ill children, all aged between eight and 14 years and attending public schools in Long Island, New York, were tested on the Rorschach, Brown Personality Inventory and Despert Fables. The cardiac children had a significantly greater total neurotic score (Brown Personality Inventory) and gave significantly more dependent responses (Despert Fables) than normal children, matched for age, sex, socio-economic group, religion and number of siblings. Asthmatic children were more maladjusted (Rorschach), neurotic (Brown Personality Inventory) and dependent (Despert Fables) than their matched normal controls. Significant differences were not found between the asthmatic and the cardiac children. Nor were there any significant differences between the chronically ill children and their healthy siblings. Findings suggest that children with a chronic illness have an emotional pattern that differs from the normal. The similar personality pattern in the siblings may be due to constitutional factors or to the presence of a chronically ill child in the family.

2 REED, M.K. (1959)

'The intelligence, social maturity, personal adjustment, physical development, and parent-child relationships of children with congenital heart disease', *Dissertation Abstracts*, 20, Part I, 385.

Fifty children with congenital heart disease, aged three to eight years, attending a cardiac out-patient clinic, did not differ significantly from non-handicapped controls (matched for age, sex, socio-economic status and number of siblings) in intelligence (Binet scale), social maturity (Vineland scale) or personal adjustment (clinically assessed). The severity of the defect was not related to intelligence or social maturity. Subjective impressions suggested that the children with heart defects had greater social anxiety and perceptiveness and were more eager to please the examiner, while the non-handicapped children were more relaxed. Mothers of girls with congenital heart defects scored significantly higher than mothers of the non-handicapped girls on scales of 'intrusiveness' and 'fostering dependency' (Parental Attitude Research Instrument), but there were no significant differences between the mothers of boys in the two groups. Most mothers of the cardiac children seemed to have made a fairly realistic adjustment, and to have made good use of the medical advice given at the clinic.

3 STEARNS, S, (1959)

'Self-destructive behaviour in young patients with diabetes mellitus', *Diabetes*, 8, 5, 379—82.

The author suggests that patterns of unreasonable behaviour found in many young diabetics, such as the purposeful omission of food or overdosage of insulin to produce hypoglycaemia, are best understood as self-destructive. The treatment and possible complications of diabetes give the young diabetic the means for acting out the self-destructive behaviour. Such behaviour occurs most frequently at critical periods of adjustment when the young diabetic feels hopeless and worthless. Where parents are unable to handle their own feelings about the diabetic child and become rejecting or hostile or where economic circumstances are poor such behaviour is more likely to occur. The patient must gently and gradually be brought to a realistic understanding of his illness as soon as such behaviour appears — if it is allowed to become established treatment is very difficult. Parents may need to be helped with their own problems before they can help the young diabetic.

4 BROWNE, W.J., MALLY, M.A. and KANE, R.P. (1960)

'Psychosocial aspects of hemophilia; a study of twenty-eight hemophilic children and their families', *American Journal of Orthopsychiatry*, 30, 4, 730—40.

A study of the effect on the course of the illness of emotional factors and mother-child relationships. Twenty-eight haemophiliac children aged one to 16 attending a clinic in Pittsburgh were interviewed or observed, and their medical histories studied; parents were also interviewed. Only a minority of bleeding episodes were apparently precipitated by injuries, although injuries were more frequent on specific occasions, suggesting accident-proneness. Generally, spontaneous bleeding was more common, and appeared to show a seasonal variation, occurring most often at Christmas or other holiday times or whenever the child was anticipating some activity or increased independence. Personality patterns as assessed by Rorschach tests indicated conflict and aggression underlying docility. Parents reacted to the diagnosis of haemophilia with anxiety and unhappiness, and mothers felt particular guilt at being carriers of the disease, which seemed to result in more over-protectiveness than is found in mothers of children with other handicaps.

5 DOWLING, J.P. (1960)

'Preventing dependency patterns in chronically ill children', *Social Casework*, 41, 8, 395—402.

Necessities of protecting haemophiliac children from many every-day dangers may mean that the mother comes to provide all controls for the child herself, or with other adults, and does not let him play his own part in determining behaviour limits. The result is that some haemophiliacs become entirely dependent on the mother or other adults. The beginnings of dependent behaviour were found in five children and three adolescents hospitalized for periods of two months to a year or more as subjects of a long-term medical study into haemophilia. The author describes the measures used by the physician, nursing staff and social worker to prevent the development of passive behaviour: (1) giving the children factual information about the illness; (2) helping the children to separate feelings of badness and low self-esteem from the necessities of the illness which require restrictions and painful procedures; (3) helping the children to participate in their own management; (4) providing a permissive setting in the hospital and letting the children test out the greater freedom.

6 LANDTMAN, B., VALANNE, E.H., PENTTI, R. and AUKEE, M. (1960)

'Psychosomatic behaviour of children with congenital heart disease. Pre- and post-operative studies of 84 cases', *Annales Paediatriac Fenniae*, 6, Supplement 15, 78pp.

A study of the psychosomatic behaviour of 84 Finnish children with congenital heart disease, aged five to 17 years, before and after heart surgery. The children represented socially a cross-section of the Finnish population. The child's closest relative (mothers in 74 cases) was interviewed by the medical social worker on the child's admission to hospital; all the children were given a battery of psychological tests when they were settled in hospital and awaiting the operation. Follow-up studies were carried out three months and one year after the operation. Improvements in exercise tolerance (63 children), appetite (47), sleep habits (42) susceptibility to infections (48) were found after the operation. Cardiological studies showed that the results were good in all cases. Before the operation 39 children were within the normal intelligence range (90—109), while 21 were below and 19 above. After the operation 23 children increased by more than 10 points, while only four children decreased by this amount. Increase in intelligence was not related to increase of exercise ability or increased oxygen supply to the brain. The greatest improvement was found in children whose behaviour and emotional environment also changed favourably. Personality traits, such as concentration, endurance, and self-confidence were generally in the average range before the operation and did not change significantly afterwards.

Before the operation, though, 36 children showed signs of stress proness, but this disappeared or diminished after the operation. Responses to Rosenzweig's frustration test did not differ significantly from those found in a study of normal Finnish children (Takala and Takala, 1955) and although there were departures from the American norms these were not in a consistent direction. Any changes after the operation tended to be in the direction of the normal. Before the operation 37 mothers were considered to be normal in their attitudes to the child, 25 over-protective and eight rejecting. After the operation no changes were found in the attitudes of mothers considered normal, but improvements occurred in 11 over-protective and four rejecting mothers. In 46 cases the mothers reported that the children showed behaviour disturbances before the operation (mainly temper tantrums and disturbed sleep). In most of these cases mothers were over-protective or the family background was unfavourable. Thirty-seven of these children showed improvements after the operation, probably due in many cases to the change in the mothers' attitudes. Only three children appeared to be anxious or fearful on the day of the operation itself and only three did not like returning to the hospital for post-operative checks. This difference from studies reporting that hospitals are upsetting for children and may have long-term adverse effects was possibly due to having a special ward for children with heart disease, to the attention paid by the staff to the children's emotional needs and to the children's familiarity with the hospital from previous visits to the cardiac clinic.

7 WEIL, W.B. Jr. and SUSSMAN, M.B. (1961)

'Behaviour, diet and glucosuria of diabetic children in a summer camp', *Pediatrics*, 27, 1, 118—27.

In a dietary experiment at a summer camp for diabetic children it was found that there was an increase of glucose in the urine (glucosuria) but fewer insulin reactions (hypoglycaemia) when the boys were on a self-regulated diet (boys chose as much as they wished from an offered menu) than when they were on a prescribed diet (insulin dosage was maintained at the level prescribed for each boy by his own physician throughout the experiment). Until it is known whether increased glucosuria or increased hypoglycaemia is the more harmful it cannot be said which dietary programme was the better — but the effects produced by the diets could be changed by altering the insulin dosages or the level of food intake. Boys judged to be well adjusted by the camp staff experienced a 22 per cent increase in glucosuria during the self-regulated diet period compared with 71 per cent increase in the boys judged to be poorly adjusted. This could, partly, but not entirely, be attributed to a greater increase in food intake in the poorly adjusted group. Psychological factors probably were responsible for part of the increase—previous studies have shown a relationship between emotional stress and increased glucosuria. The increased food intake of the poorly adjusted group may also have been due to psychological stress — a relationship between overeating and emotional disturbance has also been demonstrated in previous research.

8 ALBY, J.M. ALBY, N. and CAEN, J. (1962)

'Problèmes psychologiques de l'hémophile' ('Psychological problems in haemophilia'), *Nouvelle Revue Francaise d'Hématologie*, 2, 1, 119—30.

A discussion of the problems of haemophiliac patients and their parents and the doctor's role in relation to these. Restrictions, whether necessary or excessive, can lead to passivity or agressive opposition. Anxiety about bleeding is inevitable, and as the child is usually taken to hospital with each haemorrhage he is separated from the needed love and reassurance of his parents. Adaptation to the illness is most successful where the child can mobilize his intellectual abilities to compensate for the physical restriction. The mother's knowledge that genetic transmission is through her usually gives rise to guilt, whether conscious or unconscious and can lead to recriminations and estrangement between the parents. The mother's realistic anxiety about her child's condition is heightened by her guilt so that she becomes unable to allow the child to incur reasonable risks. It is rare to find maternal rejection of a haemophiliac child. The hospital specialist is usually the key figure for the patient and his family — their psychological dependence on him should be recognized. Nevertheless they should be given full information about the illness so that they can cope for themselves whenever possible.

9 ETZWILER, D.D. and SINES, L.K. (1962)

'Juvenile diabetes and its management: family, social and academic implications', *Journal of the American Medical Association*, 181, 304—8.

Medical, family, social and academic information about 72 diabetic children (aged six to 15 years), mainly from middle-income families, attending a summer camp, was obtained from parents, physicians, school teachers and camp counsellors. Mothers were found to play the major role in the management of the disease, taking the child to the physician, preparing the diet, administering the insulin (in 80·6 per cent of cases) and testing the urine (45·8 per cent). Most children (88·7 per cent) took some part in urine testing but only a third were involved in administering the insulin. It is suggested that the child should not assume primary responsibility for the management of his illness until he has a good understanding of the condition. Knowledge of the illness (only 15 per cent of children and 33 per cent of parents could answer 14 out of 15 basic questions about diabetes) and management practices need to improve if the incidence of long-term complications is to be minimized.

10 FEINSTEIN, A.R., TAUBE, H., CAVALIERI, R., SCHULTZ, S.C. and KRYLE, L. (1962)

'Physical activities and rheumatic heart disease in asymptomatic patients', *Journal of the American Medical Association*, 180, 12, 1028—31.

Limitation of physical activities at school, outside school or in the post-school years had no beneficial effects on the cardiac status of subjects who had rheumatic heart disease (mainly without clinical symptoms), but it did have adverse psychological consequences. Of 141 subjects who had been restricted at school 24 per cent improved in cardiac status over a five-year or longer period, 62 per cent remained the same and 14 per cent deteriorated; of the 75 subjects who had not been restricted at school, 21 per cent improved, 71 per cent remained the same and eight per cent became worse. Adverse psychosocial consequences were found in 34 per cent of the subjects who had been restricted in physical activities at school but in only 6 per cent of those who had not been restricted. Psychosocial effects were not significantly related to changes in cardiac status. Subjects (average age 30·9) were patients who attended an out-patient clinic at the New York University School of Medicine for an annual check-up.

11 GREEN, M. and LEVITT, E.E. (1962)

'Constriction of body image in children with congenital heart disease', *Pediatrics*, 29, 438—41.

Self-drawings of 25 children with congenital heart disease (aged eight to 16 years) were significantly smaller than the self-drawings of 25 normal children, matched by age and sex. The self-drawings of the normal subjects were also significantly taller than their drawings of peers, while the heights of self- and peer-drawings in the cardiac group were almost identical. Previous research has shown that there is a slight negative correlation between the size of figure drawings and the subject's own estimate of his size, so the results cannot be explained by the relatively smaller physical size of the cardiac children. Further investigation is necessary to determine why children with congenital heart disease have, in general, a constricted view of their bodies.

12 TREUTING, T.F. (1962)

'The role of emotional factors in the etiology and course of idabetes mellitus: a review of recent literature', *American Journal of the Medical Sciences*, 244, 1, 131—47.

Four areas are reviewed: (1) Role of psychological factors in the aetiology of diabetes — the research suggests that sustained and chronic emotional conflict may be a factor in the onset of the illness;

(2) Role of psychological factors in the course of the illness — fluctuations in the course of diabetes — expressed by ketonemia, an increased excretion of glucose, water and chlorides or alterations of blood glucose levels have been found to be related to emotional factors, although exactly how and why is not known for certain. The type of emotional stress producing these fluctuations differs for different patients. These changes are more important and frequent in juvenile diabetes; (3) Attitudes and reactions produced by the illness — most researchers emphasize the uniqueness of diabetes amongst chronic illness, special characteristics include its frequently asymptomatic character in the early years, the necessity for diet, insulin injections and urinanalysis, the stigma of diabetes and feeling it gives of being apart from other people, the knowledge of possible later complications and anxiety about this, and the active responsibility of the patient for control of the disease. All these features may give rise to emotional problems, particularly in the young patient. A child with diabetes often uses the illness and its management as a weapon if relationships with the parents are disturbed; (4) Role of psychological factors in treatment — effective control of diabetes requires the co-operation of the patient and the physician needs to understand him as a person.

13 DANOWSKI, T.S. (1963)

'Emotional stress as a cause of diabetes mellitus', *Diabetes*, 12, 2, 183—4.

Reconsideration of the problem leads to the conclusion that emotional stress cannot cause diabetes in normal individuals but it may bring about clinical manifestations of the illness in those who have an inherent predisposition to diabetes.

14 GOLDY, F.B. and KATZ, A.H. (1963)

'Social adaptation in hemophilia', *Children*, 10, 189—93.

Findings are reported from an investigation of 1,100 adult haemophiliacs, carried out by the University of California at Los Angeles. Forty subjects, selected to represent those who had made relatively good or poor social adjustment, were interviewed in order to explore the relationship between early childhood experiences and later adjustment. Subjects generally felt that their mothers had been over-protective — whether or not the mothers knew they were carriers of the disease. Over-protection, though, was accepted from mothers but not from fathers. The key factor in the haemophiliac's achievement of social competence and independence was his father's attitude — 'good adjusters' had fathers who were permissive or indifferent while 'poor adjusters' were over-protected by both parents. Whether the haemophiliac felt himself to be different from others depended not on the severity of his illness but on whether he had been allowed to take part in normal play with other children. A large number of 'good adjusters' said that their parents had encouraged normal childhood activities while most of the 'poor adjusters' had experienced parental opposition. Subjects thought that parents of haemophiliac children should allow the child himself to learn his own limits. Adolescence was often less difficult than earlier childhood for the haemophiliac because there were bases for social relationships other than physical activities. The authors conclude that counselling should be available to parents from the time of the diagnosis so that they can be helped to provide an environment which will encourage development and independence in the children. (See also Katz, 1963, below).

15 KATZ, A.H. (1963)

'Social adaptation in chronic illness; a study of hemophilia', *American Journal of Public Health*, 53, 10, 1666—75.

Findings from a questionnaire survey of 1,055 haemophiliac adults from all over the United States are reported and discussed (see Goldy and Katz, 1963, for a report of the second part of this study). Seventy-six point nine per cent of the sample had experienced arthropathies (joint stiffening or haemophilic arthritis — the usual cause of disabilities among haemophiliacs) at some time, but only just over half had received rehabilitative care for them, although recent medical advances have made it possible to correct arthropathies, especially if identified and treated early. About six per cent of the sample, generally, but by no means always, severely handicapped, had rarely or never worked. Such individuals also often had limited social participation and did not contemplate marriage. The author considers that they have never established a self-concept as a social competent individual who has the limiting condition of haemophilia; instead their self-concept is of a chronically handicapped person. Many haemophiliacs though, have a strong drive towards as normal a social role as possible — in work, marriage and other social relationships. Forty-nine per cent of the sample were or had been married. Fifty-two point one per cent were employed — many in jobs involving physical work — 1·14 per cent were retired and 26·4 per cent still at school. The income level of those employed was similar to that in the general population. Among the measures recommended to help more haemophiliacs to lead satisfactory lives are parental counselling, early medical treatment to prevent impairments and earlier vocational counselling.

16 STERKY, G. (1963)

'Family background and state of mental health in a group of diabetic schoolchildren', *Acta Paediatrica* (Stockholm), 52, 377—90.

One hundred and nineteen diabetic school-children

(aged seven to 20 years), living in Stockholm, were paired with 119 non-diabetic children on the basis of sex, age, school class and employment of father; the children were observed over the period of a year during a number of physical examinations and their mothers were interviewed. A much higher rate of mental disturbance was found among the mothers of the diabetics (27·6 per cent) than among the mothers of the non-diabetic children (11·1 per cent), the most common disturbance in both groups being anxiety. Among the children, mental disturbance was absent in as many diabetics (54·5 per cent) as non-diabetics (55·6 per cent). When diabetic children did show mental disturbance, however, they tended to have more symptoms than the mentally disturbed non-diabetic children. Emotional lability and difficulties with companions were found significantly more often among the mentally disturbed diabetic children than among the non-diabetic. Most of the mental disorders were mild, but five diabetics and one non-diabetic child had severe disorders. School achievements were similar in the diabetics and non-diabetics. No connection was found between school-achievement and age of onset of diabetes, duration or diabetic control. Diabetic children with mental disturbance were more likely than those without to have mentally disturbed mothers or poor diabetic control.

17 AGLE, D.P. (1964)

'Psychiatric studies of patients with hemophilia and related states', *Archives of Internal Medicine*, 114, 76—82.

A report of findings from psychiatric interviews with 16 subjects (13 with haemophilia, three with Christmas disease). All subjects felt a realistic fear of the bleeding, and resulting pain and separation from their families. A prominent feeling in childhood was fear of immobility. Nine subjects thought they had experienced extreme over-protection from their mothers (although the fathers often showed little interest in them). Not being allowed to take part in normal childhood activities had emphasized their feelings of difference from other children. Over-protection and fear of activity led to two extremes of behavioural response — recurrent risk-taking (seen in nine subjects who reported extreme over-protection) or passive dependent behaviour (seen in two subjects). In eight other cases subjects reported that their behaviour had changed from passive dependence to a more aggressive independence and that there had been a subsequent improvement in their clinical state (verified by objective evidence in five cases). It was also reported (by ten subjects) that episodes of spontaneous bleeding sometimes followed stressful emotional situations or the anticipation of such situations. The study suggests that psychological factors may affect the course of the illness. Counselling the parents so that they allow reasonable activities in childhood might prevent some of the psychological problems which have an adverse effect on the illness from arising.

18 RICHARDSON, S.A., HASTORF, A.H. and DORNBUSCH, S.M. (1964)

'Effects of physical disability on a child's description of himself', *Child Development*, 35, 3, 893—907.

One hundred and seven handicapped (handicaps included cerebral palsy, diabetes, cardiac disorders and orthopaedic disabilities) and 128 non-handicapped nine-to 11-year-old New York children at a summer camp for disadvantaged children were interviewed and asked to tell about themselves. The handicapped children shared the high value placed on physical activities by other children in their age group but they were realistic about their own abilities. They appeared to experience impoverishment in social relationships both within and outside the family. They tended to be less confident and more self-deprecatory than the non-handicapped children.

19 SCHIFF, L.J. (1964)

'Emotional problems of diabetic children and their parents', *Psychosomatics*, 5, 6, 362—4.

At the onset of diabetes parents almost always have feelings of guilt. Some parents refuse to accept the diagnosis; others regard the illness as an unwelcome burden. Over-protection, often an outcome of rejection, may produce either a rebellious or a completely dependent child. Faulty parental attitudes are likely to lead to difficulties in the management of diabetes. The severe regimentation of life required for the control of diabetes can be very trying for the parents. Some diabetics use the illness as a weapon to punish themselves or others or to gain sympathy. In adolescence the young person may associate abandonment of the diabetic regimen with emancipation from parental control. Parents and doctors must be prepared to tolerate some experimentation and irregularity or they may make matters worse. In adolescence, too, the young person begins to think seriously about employment, marriage and parenthood. Personal and vocational counselling are necessary.

20 SWIFT, C.R. and SEIDMAN, F.L. (1964)

'Adjustment problems of juvenile diabetes', *Journal of the American Academy of Child Psychiatry*, 3, 3, 500—15.

In this pilot investigation of the emotional aspects of juvenile diabetes 40 children and young adults (ages two to 20), referred by private physicians in the New Jersey area, were given a psychiatric interview and a battery of psychological tests; parents were interviewed by a psychiatric social worker. 62·5 per cent of the children were judged by the psychiatrist and psychologist to be normal and 37·5 per cent to be pathological. Prominent features of the group were greater manifest anxiety than would be expected for age (in 52·5 per cent), greater latent anxiety (85 per cent), greater oral preoccupation (preoccupation with food) (50 per cent) and a damaged or inadequate body image (55 per cent). While 40 per cent of the children were more dependent than would be expected for their age ten per cent were more independent. The social worker judged the emotional tone of the home to be good in 67·5 per cent of cases. Mothers acceptance of the disease was realistic in 71·7 per cent of cases but 48·7 per cent of mothers were overprotective and 10·3 per cent neglectful. Control of the diabetes was good in 37·5 per cent of cases and poor in 17·5 per cent. 52·5 per cent of the children showed good over-all adjustment (at home, at school, with peers), 35 per cent fair and 12·5 per cent poor. Control of diabetes was better in children who were well adjusted, classified as normal by the psychiatrist, showed less anxiety and had a better body image; it was also better where the emotional tone of the home was good and the diabetes less severe and of shorter duration. The less severe the illness the better the school adjustment and over-all adjustment. Socio-economic status was significantly related to over-all adjustment and psychiatric evaluation. While this group of diabetic children had a high proportion of adjustment problems the authors also found that many showed remarkable personality strengths — as with other continuing stresses, diabetes may give rise to adjustment or emotional difficulties in children who are susceptible, but may accelerate maturity in others.

21 DAVIS, D.M., SHIPP, J.C. and PATTISHALL, E.G. (1965)

'Attitudes of diabetic boys and girls towards diabetes', *Diabetes*, 14, 2, 106—9.

Fifty-eight 8-to 15-year-old diabetic children (average duration of the diabetes 5·1 years) attending a Florida camp for diabetic children were interviewed to investigate their attitudes towards the illness. Findings suggest that diabetic children do not feel that the illness limits their educational, occupational or marital opportunities. The children studied did not think that diabetes was much of a handicap in their daily lives, only 33 per cent feeling it interfered with their eating and 23 per cent with school activities. The majority of the children said they preferred having diabetes to other conditions, even less serious ones such as acne or obesity. The authors conclude that the children accepted diabetes as part of their lives, but did not fully understand the seriousness of their condition.

22 KATZ, A.H. (1966)

'Living with haemophilia', *New Society*, 18 August, 260—2.

Another report of the study of 1,055 adult haemophiliacs in the United States (see also Goldy and Katz, 1963; Katz, 1963). A comparison was made between the 'unsuccessful' subjects (about 14 per cent of the haemophiliacs who had left school — those who were over 25 years of age and chronically unemployed) and the 'successful' group (those over 25 years of age and employed). Haemophiliacs in the unsuccessful group were more often (but not invariably) severely affected by the illness, were less likely to be married, to have completed secondary school or to have an active social life. They had generally been in unskilled occupations. It is suggested that the factor of prime importance in determining the haemophiliac's social competence and independence in adult life is the father's attitude to him in childhood — fathers of the 'successful' group were reported as being permissive and supportive while fathers of the 'unsuccessful group' were over-protective. The child expected his mother to be over-protective but if his father was also over-protective his difference from other children was emphasized and he grew up with a damaged self-image.

23 LINDE, L.M., RASOF, B., DUNN, O.J. and RABB, E. (1966)

'Attitudinal factors in congenital heart disease', *Pediatrics*, 38, 1, 92—101.

A comparison of the relationship between adjustment and parental attitudes in cardiac and normal children. Subjects were 98 children with a congenital heart defect and cyanosis, 100 children with a congenital heart defect but no cyanosis, 81 healthy siblings of the cardiac children and 40 normal children. The cardiac children were significantly lower in intelligence than both the groups of normal children (Cattell Infant Scales or Revised Stanford Binet). While intelligence was unrelated to the child's adjustment or maternal attitudes in the normal children there was some relationship between these three variables in the cardiac children. There was little difference between the cardiac and normal children (both groups) in level of adjustment. Maternal attitudes were a more important determinant of the cardiac child's adjustment than the degree of his incapacity. The presence of a heart condition in the child, rather than the severity of the defect, appeared to be the main determinant of maternal anxiety. Protectiveness and attention were much greater for the cardiac child than for his healthy sibling, the sibling receiving less than the other normal children. (See also Rasof *et al.*, 1967 and Linde *et al.*, 1970).

24 MATTSSON, A. and GROSS, S. (1966a)

'Adaptational and defensive behaviour in young hemophiliacs and their parents', *American Journal of Psychiatry*, 122, 12, 1349—56.

Another account of the research reported in Mattsson and Gross (1966b), containing some additional descriptive material.

25 MATTSSON, A. and GROSS, S. (1966b)

'Social and behavioural studies on hemophilic children and their families', *Journal of Pediatrics*, 68, 952—64.

Thirty-five haemophiliac boys, from 22 families, mainly in the middle socio-economic range, were given psychiatric interviews and were observed over a two year period. Twenty-seven (77 per cent) of the boys were judged to be well-adapted to their illness. They generally took as much part as possible in sports and games with their friends, co-operated well with parents and hospital staff during bleeding episodes and had a basic understanding of their illness. Mothers of these children were able to make a good or satisfactory adjustment, despite anxiety and guilt at the time of diagnosis which often continued for several years. They were able to bring the children up with realistic restrictions, to co-operate with medical care and to explain the illness to the haemophiliac children and their siblings. The majority of the fathers of the well-adapted children, in a few cases after an initial depression at the time of diagnosis, took an active part in the children's care. Three of the eight poorly adapted children led restricted and dependent lives, having accepted the mother's over-protection, while the other five children showed recurrent risk-taking behaviour, rebelling against the anxiety of mothers who had experienced fatalities from haemophilia in their families. The study emphasizes the relationship between parental acceptance of the disease and the adjustment of the haemophiliac child. Findings in the study on the relationship of emotional stress to spontaneous bleeding and on changes in both clinical state and behaviour in adolescence are compared with those of previous research.

26 CASSELL, S. and PAUL, M.H. (1967)

'The role of puppet therapy on the emotional responses of children hospitalized for cardiac catheterization', *Journal of Pediatrics*, 71, 2, 233—9.

Twenty children (aged 3-11 years) who received puppet therapy before cardiac catheterization showed less emotional disturbance during the catheterization procedure itself and were more willing to return to the hospital for further treatment than 20 children of similar age, social class, prehospitalization problems and parental information about the catheterization, who did not receive the puppet therapy. No differences were found between the groups in emotional disturbances while still in hospital following the catheterization or after the return home, but in both groups there was a tendency towards less emotional disturbance after the hospitalization. During the puppet therapy the child and therapist acted out the catheterization procedure, with first the therapist and then the child playing the part of doctor. Puppets were realistically dressed for all the roles and miniature replicas of the catheterization equipment were used.

27 SWIFT, C.R.,
SEIDMAN, F.L. and
STEIN, H. (1967)

'Adjustment problems in juvenile diabetes', *Psychosomatic Medicine*, 29, 6, 555—71.

Fifty diabetic children (from a summer camp, clinics and private medical practices in New Jersey) and 50 control children individually matched for age, sex, grade, socio-economic status and race, were each given a psychiatric evaluation and a battery of psychological tests; parents were interviewed at home. Emotional disturbance was found much more frequently in the diabetic children (in 50 per cent) than in the controls (ten per cent). The diabetic children were found to be significantly more abnormal in dependence-independence balance, self-percepts, manifest and latent anxiety, sexual identification, hostility expression and oral preoccupation. The adjustment of the diabetic children to home and peers was significantly worse than that of the non-diabetic children: while about two-thirds of the controls were making a good adjustment only one-quarter to one-third of the diabetic children were doing so. There were no significant differences in the school adjustment of the two groups. The emotional atmosphere of the diabetic children's home was poorer and mothers showed more extreme attitudes of protection or neglect. Diabetic control became worse as the duration of the illness increased. Diabetic control was also worse in children with poorer emotional adjustment, self-percept, home adjustment and dependence-independence balance, lower IQ and family income and earlier onset of the illness. Self-percept and dependence-independence balance were related to the child's acceptance of the illness and the emotional atmosphere of the home.

28 WEIL, W.B. Jr. and
SUSSMAN, M.B. (1967)

'Social patterns and diabetic glucosuria', *American Journal of Diseases of Children*, 113, 454—60.

In an experiment at a summer camp for diabetic children it was found that groups of boys and girls, aged nine to 12 years, increased their glucosuria (excretion of glucose in the urine) more during a period in which competitive sporting activities between groups were organized than would be expected under normal camp conditions. Children under the age of eight years, though, showed relatively little change in glucosuria during the competitive period. It would appear that younger children do not respond to any great extent to group-activities and these have little effect on the stability of their diabetic control. Older children, in contrast, are affected by group activities and the less competitive these are the greater the stability of their diabetic control. Changes in glucosuria during the period of 'inter-group competition' were not related to the social adjustment of individual children.

29 BIRKBECK, J.A.,
KLONOFF, H. and
McTAGGART, A.H.
(1968)

'Emotional disturbance in juvenile diabetics', *Diabetes*, Annual Meeting Supplement, 17, 317—8.

Twenty-eight adolescents (12 boys, 16 girls) with diabetes (average age of onset eight years, average duration 5·8 years) were interviewed in-depth by a psychiatrist and given a battery of psychological tests; parents were also interviewed in-depth. The average intelligence was 118, significantly above normal (Wechsler Intelligence scale). Ten subjects (nine girls, one boy) showed evidence of significant psychiatric disturbance. There was a strong relationship between poor diabetic control and emotional disturbance. In general, subjects showed productivity, organizational ability, wide interests and effective responses, but also many features of anxiety. On the Minnesota Multiphasic Personality Inventory 38 per cent of parents showed signs of overt disturbance.

30 GARLINGHOUSE, J.
and SHARP, L.J. (1968)

'The hemophilic child's self-concept and family stress in relation to bleeding episodes', *Nursing Research*, 17, 1, 32—7.

This study found a slight relationship between family stress (as reported by the mother) and the number of spontaneous bleeding episodes experienced by a haemophiliac child. A slight relationship was also found between the strength of the child's self-concept (as measured by the Colvin Silhouette Test) and the number of bleeding episodes. This relationship only held, though, when stresses were low. When stresses were high they tended to be associated with more bleeding episodes regardless of the strength of the child's self-concept. Subjects were 18 haemophiliac children (mainly aged nine to 14 years), attending a haemophilia centre in Seattle, Washington.

31 LANDTMAN, B.,
VALANNE, E.H. and
AUKEE, M. (1968)

'Emotional implications of heart disease. A study of 256 children with real and with 'imaginary' heart disease', *Annales Paediatriae Fenniae*, 14, 3, 71—92.

A further study of the emotional adjustment of children operated on for congenital heart disease at the Children's Hospital in Helsinki (see also Landtman *et al.*, 1960). Subjects were 200 children with congenital heart defects (164 acyanotic, 36 cyanotic), including the 84 children from the original study. Time of waiting for the operation was more than five years in 111 cases. One year after the operation all the cardiac children were able to lead normal or practically normal lives. A study was also made of the emotional adjustment of 56 children who had been mistakenly diagnosed as having a heart defect, all of whom had subjective symptoms of heart complaint (time between the original diagnosis and diagnosis of freedom from defect was more than three years in 23 cases). In the cardiac children no relationship was found between the severity of the defect and the mother's attitude, the child's behaviour before the operation or the child's intelligence. Behaviour of the children, though, was related to the mother's attitudes. Improvements attitudes occurred in 47 of the mothers considered to be over-protective (61) or rejecting (nine) before the operation. Improvements were also found in the behaviour of 80 of the 133 children considered normal before the operation and in 24 of the 67 emotionally disturbed children. Thirty of the children increased in IQ by more than ten points after the operation, while only six decreased in IQ by this amount. Two years after the operation teachers reporting on the behaviour and progress of 104 of the children found improvements in almost three-quarters. A decline in the percentage of mothers who were over-protective (from 35 per cent of 13 per cent) or who showed 'excessive fear' of the operation (from 38 per cent to 12 per cent) and of pre-operative behaviour disorders in the children (from 56 per cent to 14 per cent) was found when cases investigated during 1955-9 were compared with those seen between 1965-8. At the beginning of the period few cardiac operations had been performed at the hospital, but as the number of successful operations increased physicians were able to give parents better support, and information about cardiac operations was also spread by the Finnish mass media, thus giving parents more confidence in the treatment. Emotional reactions of the children with imaginary heart disease and their mothers were very similar to those found in children who actually had heart disease. Behaviour of the children improved in 35 cases after they were told they had a normal heart, symptoms disappeared in 42 cases and the IQ of four children improved by ten or more points. School reports of these children were generally above average both before and after they were found to be free of heart disease. Four mothers could not be convinced at first that the child did not have a heart defect — the longer the mother had been under the impression that the child had a defect the more difficult it was for her attitudes to change.

32 COLLIER, B.N. Jr. (1969a)

'Comparisons between adolescents with and without diabetes', *Personnel and Guidance Journal*, 47, 679—84.

Self-descriptions of 125 diabetic adolescents attending high schools in Minnesota were found to be similar to those of non-diabetic adolescents attending the same schools. While some individuals in both groups did show maladaptive behaviour traits the number who did so was no greater than would be expected in a broad sample of adolescents.

33 COLLIER, B.N. Jr. (1969b)

'Interpersonal traits of secondary school adolescents with and without diabetes', *Rehabilitation Counseling Bulletin*, 13, 2, 190—6.

Another account of the research summarized in Collier (1969a).

34 GALDSTON, R, and GAMBLE, W.J. (1969)

'On borrowed time: observations on children with implanted cardiac pacemakers and their families', *American Journal of Psychiatry*, 126, 1, 104—8.

From observations and interviews over a seven-year period it was found that neither the 16 children and two adults, who had internal pacemakers implanted at the Children's Hospital Medical Centre, Boston, Massachussets, nor their parents, showed the signs of emotional disturbance which might have been expected. Stress on the parents and child included constant threat of failure of circulation to maintain consciousness or even life; need for frequent surgical procedures (on average at 5·6 months intervals for 12 patients) for revisions. Nevertheless, the family was able to meet the situation with relative calm, primarily by sharing the doctor's belief in medical advances — and also by taking an intellectual interest in the cardiac condition and pacemaker, by displacing worries onto relatively minor problems or dissipating them on routine care, by the use of humour, and by the strengthening of family ties around the common belief.

35 SPENCER, R.F. and BEHAR, L. (1969)

'Adaptation in hemophiliac adolescents', *Psychosomatics*, 10, 5, 304—9.

From a study of ten haemophiliac adolescents it is suggested that despite apparently good superficial adjustment many young haemophiliacs have behavioural problems, learning difficulties and sexual disturbances. The problems can be related to the haemophiliac's difficulties in the achievement of stable male identification. Case histories illustrate the argument.

36 BAKER, L. and BARCAI, A. (1970)

'Psychosomatic aspects of diabetes mellitus', in O.W. Hill (Ed.) *Modern trends in psychosomatic medicine 2*. London, Butterworths, pp. 105—23.

A critical review of the literature on the relationship between emotional factors and diabetes that is particularly concerned with the role of emotional factors in the course and control of diabetes. Previous studies of subjects with 'excessive lability' or frequent bouts of ketoacidosis have failed to differentiate between those who 'use' the diabetic state as a weapon and deliberately fail to keep to the diabetic regimen and those who suffer from ketoacidosis despite conscientious adherence to the diabetic regimen. The terms 'stress' and 'emotional arousal' have also been used imprecisely in these studies. Recent research by the present authors, using the latest knowledge concerning the role of the free fatty acids in energy metabolism, has enabled them to differentiate a sub-group of juvenile diabetics, the 'super labile' group, in whom there is a relationship between 'emotional arousal', increase in free fatty acid concentration and diabetic acidosis. A classificatory system of psychosomatic disorders in juvenile diabetes is presented by the authors.

37 GRAHAM, P. and RUTTER, M. (1970)

'Psychiatric aspects of physical disorder', in M. Rutter, J. Tizard and K. Whitmore (Eds.) *Education, health and behaviour*. London, Longman, pp. 309—27.

In a survey of handicapped children on the Isle of Wight, ten-to 12-year-old children with physical disorders (orthopaedic, heart disease, diabetes and other disorders) were found to have only a slightly higher rate of psychiatric problems (10·5 per cent), as judged from a parental questionnaire, than the general population (6·8 per cent) (difference only bordered on statistical significance). Findings were similar on a teachers' questionnaire. While significantly more of the children with physical disorders were miserable or had frequent headaches compared with the general population, rates of other behaviour difficulties were similar in the two groups.

38 KATZ, A.H. (1970a)

Hemophilia. A study in hope and reality. Springfield, Illinois, Charles C. Thomas. (Chapter 4. 'The hemophiliac's family: a total involvement').

A review of research by the author himself and by others of the emotional problems of the haemophiliac boy and his parents. The author concludes that, on the whole, his research shows that most haemophiliacs and their families have done very well, without having received much professional help or counselling — but if such help were available they could do even better and could avoid much distress.

39 KRONES, P.D. (1970)

'Level of aspiration and the evaluation of self and others by diabetic and non-diabetic children', *Dissertation Abstracts International*, 30, 8-B, 3870—1.

Forty-four children, aged ten to 16 years, attending a summer camp for diabetic children and 44 non-handicapped school-children in the same age range were administered a level of aspiration task (a modification of Rotter's level of aspiration board) and a questionnaire designed to evaluate self-concept. Significantly more of the diabetic, than of the non-diabetic children, were found to over-estimate or under-estimate their ability on the level of aspiration task — indicating that the diabetic child has negative feelings about himself more frequently than the non-diabetic child. No other significant differences were found between the two groups, although the diabetic children had been more anxious, concerned at being like other children and more liable to misunderstand instructions in the experimental situation.

40 LaHOOD, B.J. (1970)

'Parental attitudes and their influence on the medical management of diabetic adolescents', *Clinical Pediatrics*, 9, 8, 468—71.

Juvenile diabetics, previously in good medical control, may experience repeated episodes of acidosis in adolescence. Many factors, including metabolic disturbances, susceptibility to infection and emotional disturbances have been suggested as being responsible. In some cases, though, the diabetic adolescent deliberately sabotages his medical regimen. He is most likely to be rebelling against the over-protective attitudes of his parents, which arise from their feelings of guilt and anxiety. A social worker or other professional should assess family relationships and management of the condition from the time of diagnosis, so that faulty parental attitudes can be prevented or corrected and the parents helped to shift from an earlier mode of management to one in which the adolescent is allowed more independence.

41 LINDE, L.M., RASOF, B. and DUNN, C.J. (1970)

'Longitudinal studies of intellectual and behavioural development in children with congenital heart disease', *Acta Paediatrica Scandinavica*, 59, 2, 169—176.

The final report of a series of studies over a five-year period comparing the intelligence and adjustment of children with cyanotic and acyanotic heart disease and normal children (see also Linde *et al.*, 1966; Rasof *et al.*, 1967). During this period more than 40 per cent of the cardiac children underwent operations, and the present study compares the development of operated and non-operated children. All groups made some gains in mean IQ, but the only change that reached statistical significance was in the operated cyanotic group. Initial low IQ in the cyanotic children can be attributed, at least in part, to their incapacity and the IQ increment to clinical improvement following the operation. Acyanotic children were less handicapped and nearer to their true potential and, therefore, less change occurred whether or not they were operated upon. As with intellectual change the greatest improvement in adjustment and behaviour occurred in the operated cyanotic group. The non-operated cyanotic group showed a significant decline in general adjustment, while both the operated and non-operated acyanotic groups showed no change. Mothers of operated children, cyanotic and acyanotic, decreased in anxiety and pampered and protected their children less during the study period. Mothers of the non-operated acyanotic children also decreased in protectiveness, probably due to the decline in symptoms in this group with age.

42 COLLIER, B.N. Jr. and ETZWILER, D.D. (1971)

'Comparative study of diabetes knowledge among juvenile diabetics and their parents', *Diabetes*, 20, 1, 51—7.

Children with diabetes and their parents were found to be similarly knowledgeable about the illness. Subjects — 129 diabetic children from 58 junior and senior high schools in the Minneapolis—St. Paul area and their parents — were given a 34 item test to evaluate their knowledge of diabetes. The child's knowledge was not related to parental income, educational level of the mother, grade level or duration of diabetes. Areas in which knowledge was particularly deficient were those concerning recognition of symptoms associated with the development of acidosis and those related to the understanding of diet. The authors point out that it is essential for the child and his parents to be properly informed and motivated if effective control is to be achieved.

43 DEL VECCHIO, F.A.
(1971)

'A comparative study of selected personality variables in diabetic and non-diabetic children', *Dissertation Abstracts International*, 32, 2-B, 1208.

Previous research has suggested that diabetic children are more constricted than non-handicapped children. The present study compared two possible manifestations of constriction — level of anxiety and creative ability — in 50 diabetic children (aged seven to 16 years), living in New Jersey, and 50 control children, matched for age range, sex, race, IQ, school-grade and socio-economic status. The two groups showed no overall differences in creative ability (Minnesota Test of Creative Thinking). Some evidence that the diabetic children were more anxious was found (Rorschach and Lie scale of the General Anxiety Scale for Children) (GASC), but the scores of the two groups did not differ on the GASC itself.

44 GERSTEIN, O.B.
(1971)

'The relationship between perception of parental behaviour, level of dependency and vocational interest in hemophilic young adults', *Dissertation Abstracts International*, 31, 12-A, 6401.

In this study a significant relationship was found between a haemophiliac's level of dependency (as measured by the 'tendermindedness' and 'submissiveness' factors of Scheier and Cattell's Neuroticism Scale Questionnaire, 1961) and his vocational interest pattern (Strong Vocational Interest Blank, 1943). The quality of 'tendermindedness' (as opposed to 'toughmindedness') was significantly related to the choice of a social service occupation while 'submissiveness' (as opposed to 'dominance') was significantly related to the choice of a non-social occupation. A relationship was also found between the haemophiliac's perception of parental behaviour and his vocational interest pattern, e.g. the more rewarding the mother was seen to be in ways that showed love for the child the more likely he was to choose a social service career. Contrary to the author's expectations, no significant relationship was found between the son's perception of parental behaviour and his level of dependency. It is possible that anxiety or self-concept, rather than dependency, are the intervening links between home influences and the development of vocational interests. Subjects were 60 haemophiliacs, aged 15 to 20 years, from New York city and the Delaware Valley.

45 MATTSSON, A., GROSS, S. and HALL, T.W. (1971)

'Psychoendocrine study of adaptation in young hemophiliacs', *Psychosomatic Medicine*, 33, 3, 215—25.

A study of the psychosocial functioning (as assessed by a paediatrician and a psychiatrist — areas covered were social relationships, range of physical activities, academic performance, interests, and adaptation to handicap) of ten haemophiliac boys, aged six to 14 years initially, over a three-year period. The relationship of psychosocial functioning to adrenal cortical activity, which previous research has shown to be sensitive to psychologic influences, (as measured by the urinary 17 OHCS excretions) was investigated in three situations — at home, during in-patient stays at the research centre and when hospitalized for the care of acute haemorrhages — and, contrary to the authors' expectations, high adaptation was found to be significantly related to high 17 OHCS excretions (indicating relatively high psychological arousal). As was expected, the boys with higher adaptation had higher barrier scores on Holtzman's Inkblot test (i.e. they had a higher number of responses emphasizing a surface or covering — it is assumed that the barrier score relates to the individual's perception of his body boundary as being well-defined and protective, a high score, therefore, indicating good adjustment).

46 OLCH, D. (1971a)

'Personality characteristics of hemophiliacs', *Journal of Personality Assessment*, 35, 1, 72—9.

Forty-five haemophiliacs from Seattle, Washington (see also Olch, 1971b) were administered a number of projective tests (Rorschach, draw-a-person, and making up stories to four verbal cues). Personality characteristics resembled those that have been reported for diabetics and asthmatics. Nevertheless a single typical haemophiliac personality was not found — individuals reacted to and coped with the illness in many different ways.

47 STEIN, S.P. and CHARLES, E. (1971)

'Emotional factors in juvenile diabetes mellitus: a study of early life experience of adolescent diabetics', *American Journal of Psychiatry*, 128, 6, 700—4.

This study suggests that some individuals are physiologically susceptible to diabetes and that psychological stress, such as parental loss or severe family disturbance may lead to the disease becoming clinically manifest. Sixty-nine per cent of adolescent diabetics, from a lower socio-economic level background, attending the diabetic clinic at the Bronx

Hospital Municipal Centre had suffered parental loss (due to separation, divorce or death) or severe family disturbance (severe physical or mental illness of a parent or intense marital discord), compared with 19 per cent of the control subjects, adolescents with hereditary blood disorders, from a similar social background, attending another clinic at the Hospital Centre. Seventy-seven per cent of the diabetics had suffered the parental losses before the disease was clinically diagnosed.

48 MEYERS, R.D. *et al.*, (1972)

'The social and economic impact of hemophilia — a survey of 70 cases in Vermont and New Hampshire', *American Journal of Public Health*, 62, 530—5.

A study of all the haemophiliacs who could be located in Vermont and New Hampshire. A correlation was found between the severity of the disorder and intra-family strain but strains sometimes occurred even where the illness was mild. Understanding of the illness alleviated tensions. in the families of mild haemophiliacs but could not prevent fears in the families of the severely affected. Conflict over sports activities was common between parents and the haemophiliac children, particularly where the child was severely affected. Lack of advice from their physician often resulted in parents being unnecessarily restrictive. Only six of the haemophiliacs who were of school-age or over were not receiving or had not received their education within the public school system. Schools, though, like parents tended to place unnecessary restrictions on the child. Only one haemophiliac in the sample had received vocational guidance. Fifty-five per cent of the adults had experienced some difficulty in their present employment because of their illness. Improvements in vocational guidance, family planning advice and cover of medical expenses are necessary if the problems of the haemophiliac are to be eased.

49 TIETZ, W. and VIDMAR, J.T. (1972)

'The impact of coping styles on the control of juvenile diabetes', *Psychiatry in Medicine*, 3, 1, 67—74.

In this study of 21 children with diabetes, from a lower socio-economic level background (15 from minority ethnic groups), no correlation was found between the degree of control of diabetes and its duration, knowledge of diabetes, number of siblings, intactness of family, degree of psychopathology, intelligence of the child or parents, birth rank, ethnic group or social class. A relationship between good control and a family history of diabetes was found. A number of those with only fair or poor control appeared to be in the midst of an adolescent growth spurt, suggesting that biological factors may play a part in control. The onset of the diabetes had a great impact on all the families. The initial shock was followed by a basic anxiety that the child might die. This fear was often partially repressed but persisted on a preconscious or conscious level. It is suggested that the family style of coping with this fear affects the degree of control achieved. The argument is illustrated with case studies.

SECTION II   Family adjustment

Research in the previous section has established that there is a close association between parental and child adjustment in all the conditions — cardiac disorders, diabetes and haemophilia — that are the concern of this review. Although the literature on these disorders contains considerable discussion on the emotional problems of the parents much is based on clinical impressions. Few studies have compared attitudes of the parents with those of parents of non-handicapped children or examined the extent of emotional problems in a representative sample of the parents.

CARDIAC DISORDERS   Only one study, a five-year investigation of the adjustment of children with congenital heart defects, carried out in the United States, actually compares attitudes of parents of cardiac children with those of parents of non-handicapped children (Linde *et al.*, 1966). Maternal protectiveness and anxiety were found to be higher in the cardiac than in the normal group. Although mothers of children with a cyanotic heart defect (producing bluish colour of lips and nailbeds) were more protective and anxious than mothers of children with heart defects but no cyanosis the difference was only slight while the cyanotic children were considerably more incapacitated physically. It is suggested that it is the presence of a heart defect rather than its severity that produces maternal anxiety. Evidence from a major study of cardiac children carried out in Finland (Landtman *et al.*, 1968) supports this view. While the greater incapacity of the cyanotic children may be a factor in their mothers' greater anxiety later findings (Linde *et al.*, 1970) suggests that the presence of the cyanosis (a visible defect) is also partly responsible.

Several studies, both British (Apley *et al.*, 1967) and American (Maxwell and Gane, 1962; Glaser *et al.*, 1964) as well as the Finnish study mentioned above (Landtman *et al.*, 1968) have been concerned with the strains on the family of a child with congenital heart disease. The most common maternal reaction to the initial diagnosis was said to be 'shock' in two studies (Apley *et al.*, 1967; Landtman *et al.*, 1968) and 'fear' in a third study (Maxwell and Gane, 1962). Some of the researchers suggest that an awareness of the vital role of the heart to life may mean that congenital heart disorder has a greater emotional impact than other serious disorders (Glaser *et al.*, 1964; Apley *et al.*, 1967; Landtman *et al.*, 1968). Apley and his associates found some evidence to support this suggestion — at outpatient clinics in the Bristol area fathers as well as mothers accompanied children with suspected heart disease on their first attendance in 50 per cent of cases, while only 17 per cent of children with other conditions were accompanied by both parents.

Delay in confirmation of the initial diagnosis had a disturbing emotional effect on the parents (Glaser *et al.*, 1964; Apley *et al.*, 1967). Apley *et al.* found that more than half of the mothers in their sample, including a third of those judged to be well-adjusted, were dissatisfied to some extent with diagnostic consultations at hospitals. Parental anxiety was partly responsible for poor communication but insufficient explanation and assurance by doctors and their concentration on the medical aspects of the child's condition added to the difficulties.

Mothers may blame themselves for the child's heart defect (Glaser *et al.*, 1964; Landtman *et al.*, 1968). Ten of the 25 mothers of cardiac children attending a Colorado clinic (Glaser *et al.*, 1964) felt themselves to be wholly responsible for the child's condition, five blaming their physical inadequacy and two, who had not wanted a child, believing that the defect was a punishment for this.

Some parents also suffer from constant anxiety that the child may suddenly die (Maxwell and Gane, 1962; Glaser *et al.*, 1964; Landtman *et al.*, 1968), although this is very unusual in most types of congenital heart defect. Parents found difficulties in disciplining the children (Maxwell and Gane, 1962; Glaser, 1964) and were often reluctant to follow the physician's advice to let the child find his own level of physical activity (Glaser *et al.*, 1964). There was also a tendency to centre attention in the family on the child with the heart defect Glaser *et al.*, 1964; Linde *et al.*, 1966; Landtman *et al.*, 1968). Linde *et al.* found that siblings of a cardiac child were less protected and pampered by their mothers than were either the cardiac children or normal children in families without a cardiac child. It is hardly surprising that 13 per cent of the siblings in one study felt jealous or deprived (Maxwell and Gane, 1962).

Major changes in family life, such as the father changing job or the family moving house occurred in

54 per cent of families in the Bristol study, social activities were restricted in 34 per cent and there were extra expenses in 45 per cent. In one of the American studies (Maxwell and Gane, 1962) 65 per cent of the families said that changes had occurred in their economic situation, social activities or parental health. Eighty-six per cent of the families in this study felt they had adjusted ('come to a reasonable acceptance of the situation, with understanding of what it implies for the future of the child and his family'), but this adjustment was judged to tenuous in some cases.

For most children with congenital heart defects the treatment is surgery. Eighty-three per cent of the parents in Maxwell and Gane's study (1962) welcomed the prospect of surgery. Landtman *et al.* (1968) found that extreme maternal anxiety about the operation became less frequent during the period of their long-term study (in which cardiac operations became much more common), diminishing from 38 per cent in mothers interviewed between 1955—9 to 12 per cent in those seen between 1965—8. Nevertheless the decision about the operation involves stress for most mothers, particularly if the child is without symptoms (Glaser *et al.*, 1964; Landtman *et al.*, 1968). Parents of a cardiac child may have to face the task of preparing the child for cardiac catheterization, which is often necessary for a definitive diagnosis, as well as the operation itself (Glaser *et al.*, 1964). Undue delay in the operation may cause over-anxiety and over-protectiveness in some parents (Apley *et al.*, 1967).

It is clear that parents of cardiac children have many common problems from the time a heart condition is first suspected. The authors of the studies discussed above point out the need for doctors to be aware of these problems and to ensure that parents are given necessary assurances and full explanations which they can understand. Landtman's study (1968) has already shown that increasing confidence in cardiac surgery has resulted not only in a reduction of excessive anxiety about the operation in mothers but also in a decrease of over-protective attitudes and in behaviour problems of the children themselves. More support and advice for parents could result in further improvements.

DIABETES

There has been much discussion on the problems of families of diabetic children but little is based on actual research evidence. Two studies which explored problems of emotional adjustment in diabetic children did, though, also consider parental adjustment (Sterky, 1963; Swift *et al.*, 1967). Sterky found a significantly higher proportion of mental disturbance in mothers of diabetic children living in Stockholm than in mothers of matched non-diabetic children, anxiety being the most frequent symptom. Swift and his associates found more turmoil and conflict in the homes of New Jersey diabetic children than in those of the matched controls. Mothers of the diabetic children also showed more extremes of attitude — either of over-protection or neglect. Another study (Crain *et al.*, 1966), particularly concerned with family functioning, found that parents of diabetic children in two areas of the United States had poorer marital relationships than those of non-diabetic children. In a recent British study (Watson, 1972) eight of the 15 parents interviewed were judged to have an 'unacceptabley high' level of anxiety and distress.

Although there is not a great deal of research on adjustment of families of diabetic children, findings do appear to consistently indicate greater parental anxiety and more conflict than in families of non-diabetics. Watson's (1972) research, which investigated the problems of a randomly selected sample from all families identified as having a diabetic child in two London boroughs, indicates some of the causes of anxiety. All parents felt shock at the diagnosis (although a few were relieved that it was not worse), and none were given an opportunity to discuss their feelings with a professional worker. Discussion at the hospitals centred on diabetic management but despite this the teaching was only fully adequate in one hospital (out of eight). Most parents felt a great anxiety about management in the first weeks at home and all felt that they lacked support (even those told they could telephone the hospital at any time). Supportive home visits would have been very much welcomed. Although most of the parents coped with management after a time nearly all were frightened about the possibility of hypoglycaemic or ketotic episodes and of the child becoming unconscious. Parents who felt that they were not in control of the child's diabetes and those who did not understand the various procedures experienced the most anxiety. In a few families life centred round the child's diabetic management. Discipline and deciding whether the child should be allowed to take part in various physical or social activities presented problems for some parents.

Many of the problems faced by parents of diabetic children then appear very similar to the problems of parents of cardiac children. The close involvement of parents in the child's management, though, and the possibility of harmful effects if this is not carried out adequately present unique features. They make it essential for parents of diabetic children to have the opportunity to discuss their fears and anxieties and to be given explanations which they fully understand.

HAEMOPHILIA

While there is no study which compares attitudes of parents of haemophiliac children with those of normal children, several researchers have been interested in the adjustment problems of parents of haemophiliacs.

Feelings of guilt in parents when they realize that their child has a congenital defect are common, as was shown by the research on parents of cardiac children discussed above. In haemophilia mothers are responsible for the genetic transmission of the illness and this appears to result in almost universal feelings of guilt on learning the diagnosis (Browne *et al.*, 1960; Alby *et al.*, 1962; Mattsson and Gross, 1966b). These feelings of guilt occur in mothers without a family history of haemophilia as well as in those with such a history (Browne *et al.*, 1960; Mattsson and Gross, 1966b).

A tendency for mothers to be over-protective and anxious is noted in several studies but it is difficult to judge from the available research how widespread this is. Browne *et al.* (1960) found all but one of the 28 mothers of haemophiliac boys attending a Pittsburgh clinic to be over-anxious and over-protective. In contrast, 16 of 22 mothers in Mattsson and Gross's (1966b) study were judged to show satisfactory or good adaptation to bring up a haemophiliac boy, although it usually took one to four years from the time of diagnosis to achieve this. All but one of the mothers who failed to make a satisfactory adaptation had had fatalities from haemophilia previously in their families.

One of the main problems for parents of haemophiliac boys is the extent to which the children should be allowed to join in physical activities with others (Browne *et al.*, 1960; Goldy and Katz, 1963; Katz, 1970a; Meyers *et al.*, 1972). Although this problem arises for parents of children with other disorders it is particularly acute for the parent of the haemophiliac. Parents may realize that haemophiliac boys need the same experiences as other children yet fear the consequences of accident. Research suggests, though, that haemophiliac children come to set their own self-limits at any early age and can protect themselves against body contact injuries (Goldy and Katz, 1963). The psychological consequences of over-protection appear to be more harmful than minor injuries (Goldy and Katz, 1963; Agle, 1964). This is a point on which parents need much guidance and reassurance from their doctors.

CONCLUSIONS

Despite the very different characteristics of cardiac conditions, diabetes and haemophilia it can be seen that parents face many of the same problems. All the conditions have features which may cause great anxiety, and possibly over-protective attitudes (although the extent of these is not clear from the research) in parents. Studies on all three conditions emphasise the need of parents for explanation, guidance and support. Recommendations made by the Working Party on children with special needs, set up under the auspices of the National Children's Bureau, (Younghusband *et al.*, 1970) that supportive services should be available to parents, are entirely upheld by the findings of these studies. The Working Party stressed that parents should be given full information about the child's condition, advice on practical care and management and an opportunity to discuss their own feelings. They pointed out that where such supportive services are lacking parents' natural concern and anxiety may turn to over-anxiety or resentment.

Abstracts

50 MAXWELL, G.M. and GANE, S. (1962)

'The impact of congenital heart disease upon the family', *American Heart Journal*, 64, 4, 449—54.

One hundred and fifty families of children with congenital heart disease, attending University Hospitals, Madison, Wisconsin, were studied, about half the group being questioned on their first visit to the clinic. Only 58 per cent had more than superficial knowledge of congenital heart disease and misconceptions as to prognosis were common. Diagnosis had usually been made before the child was five years old by the family's private physician, and 'worry', 'fright' and 'concern' were reactions in 90 per cent of the parents. Seventy-five per cent said they were satisfied with the initial consultation but 40 per cent had sought other medical advice. Fifty-nine per cent thought that care of the child gave rise to problems — discipline (50 per cent) and feeding (20 per cent) being the most common. Thirty-two per cent thought the child might suddenly die. Most (60 per cent) thought the child's condition had not affected marital relationships. Thirty-eight per cent considered that the siblings were adversely affected, mainly by worry (18 per cent) or hostility and jealously (10 per cent). Fourteen per cent of families were completely unable to 'adjust' to the situation and adjustment in some of the other families was tenuous. The majority (70 per cent) of parents reacted favourably to the possibility of surgery. Measures by which a physician can help to alleviate some of these fears and anxieties include: (1) presenting a definite diagnosis as soon as possible — and giving repeated simple explanations of this; (2) giving reassurance that the child will not suddenly die; (3) explaining that the parents are not to blame for the child's defect; (4) telling parents about the natural history of the disease so they can cope with problems as they arise, e.g. respiratory infections; (5) encouraging as much physical activity as the child's condition allows.

51 CURRAN, A.P. and McSWAN, E. (1964)

'The welfare of handicapped children. A Glasgow study' in Carnegie United Kingdom Trust, *Handicapped children and their families*. Dunfermline, T. and A. Constable, Part I, Appendix H, pp 59—65.

As part of a survey of the needs of handicapped

children and their families in the Glasgow area, 12 children with physical handicaps other than orthopaedic (five congenital heart defects, one diabetes, one Christmas disease — a form of haemophilia) were studied. Generally in this group family atmosphere was good. In only two cases were siblings adversely affected by the presence of the handicapped child, and both of these appeared to arise from faulty parental attitudes. Regular medical supervision was provided for the cardiac children and for the diabetic and the haemophiliac child. Mothers of the younger cardiac children (who were awaiting possible surgical treatment) appeared to be apprehensive and over-protective mainly because they did not understand the child's capabilities — if time could be found for answering questions at the periodic hospital assessments and if a home visitor were available to give practical guidance parental anxieties would be reduced. Housing was one of the main difficulties for families in the group. Four families of the cardiac children lived two flights up or more.

52 GLASER, H.H., HARRISON, G.S. and LYNN, D.B. (1964)

'Emotional implications of congenital heart disease in children', *Pediatrics*, 33, 367—79.

Twenty-five mothers of children with congenital heart defects (12 already operated on), attending the University of Colorado Medical Centre, were interviewed. Emotional strains on many of the mothers included: vague anxiety about the child before the diagnosis was made; lack of certainty about the child's condition even after diagnosis; fear of sudden illness or death during the child's early years; difficulties in care of an infant with poor growth and irritable temperament; centering attention on the child at the expense of the rest of the family; self-blame for the child's condition; worry about the child's ability to lead a 'normal' life; fears about permitting the physical activities advised by doctors; uncertainty over discipline; conflict of feelings about accepting recommendation for surgery; concern about the child's own fearfullness of his condition; apprehension about cardiac catheterization, the operation itself and its outcome. If the family physician is aware of these problems he can do much to alleviate them.

53 CRAIN, A.J., SUSSMAN, M.B. and WEIL, W.B. Jr. (1966a)

'Effects of a diabetic child on marital integration and related measures of family functioning', *Journal of Health and Human Behaviour*, 7, 2, 122—7.

Parents of diabetic children had significantly poorer marital relationships (as measured by goal concensus — WRU Goal Scale and Farber's Index of Marital Integration) and a tendency towards more marital conflicts (Parental Attitudes Research Instrument) and greater disagreement on how to react to the children's actions (Porter's Parental Acceptance Scale) than parents of non-diabetic children. Subjects were the middle and lower-middle class parents of 54 diabetic and 76 matched non-diabetic children. It is compatible with the findings to argue that the lower marital integration of the parents of the diabetic children could have existed before the onset of the illness and could have been an aetiological factor — previous research has suggested that disrupting family circumstances may precipitate diabetes in children who are genetically predisposed to the illness. It is more likely, though, that the lower marital integration is the outcome of the continuous crisis situation in the family caused by the diabetes.

54 CRAIN, A.J., SUSSMAN, M.B. and WEIL, W.B. Jr. (1966b)

'Family interaction, diabetes and sibling relationships', *International Journal of Social Psychiatry*, 12, 35—43.

The social-psychological functioning of diabetic children (measured by self-esteem, satisfaction with behaviour, aspiration and academic achievement) was found not to differ significantly from that of siblings of diabetic children. The social-psychological functioning of the diabetic children was closely related to the mother's behaviour but there was no similar relationship between social-psychological functioning of the non-diabetic sibling and mother's behaviour. Subjects were 19 diabetic children aged 8-11 years attending a diabetes research clinic and 16 children of similar age who had diabetic siblings attending the same clinic.

55 CUMMINGS, S.T., BAYLEY, H.C. and RIE, H.E. (1966)

'Effects of the child's deficiency on the mother: a study of mothers of mentally retarded, chronically ill and neurotic children', *American Journal of Orthopsychiatry*, 36, 4, 595—608.

Two hundred and forty mothers, 60 each with chronically physically ill children (about one-quarter diabetic, one-quarter with heart damage from rheumatic fever and one-quarter with cystic fibrosis), mentally retarded children, neurotic children and healthy children, completed five self-administered attitude tests. In comparison with mothers of the healthy children the mothers of the chronically ill children were the least deviant.

56 APLEY, J., BARBOUR, R.F. and WESTMACOTT, I. (1967)

'Impact of congenital heart disease on the family: preliminary report', *British Medical Journal*, i, 103—5.

In 88 families of children with congenital heart disease living in Bristol or the Southwest, 39 per cent of mothers were excessively disturbed by the initial 'shock' of the diagnosis. Family balance was upset (e.g. father changed job, house re-organized) in 54 per cent of the families and social activities were restricted in 36 per cent. Siblings showed behaviour problems in 27 per cent of families, psychosomatic disorders in 13 per cent and both behaviour problems and psychosomatic disorders in 24 per cent. A greater emotional impact than for other serious disorders is suggested by the father as well as the mother accompanying the child on first attendence at the paediatric outpatient clinic in 50 per cent of cases, compared with fathers being present in only 17 per cent of cases of children attending for non-cardiac conditions. Severity of the heart defect appeared to play some role in determining the impact on the family, disturbances in family life being much more common in families of 12 children with incurable cardiac conditions than in those of 12 children (not included in the series) who were declared free of any cardiac defect after some years of hospital attendance. Sixty mothers, judged to be 'specifically over-reacting' (over-protective or rejecting) were compared with 28 mothers judged to be well-adjusted — the 'specifically over-reacting' mothers were more likely to be generally immature, not satisfied with the interview, to have families in which the balance was upset, to be prone to anxiety, to be excessively upset by the diagnosis, to have a restricted social life; they were less likely to leave the child with neighbours or let the siblings play normally with him. Delays and uncertainty in confirmation of the diagnosis and delay in the operation were associated with over-anxiety and disturbance in family patterns. Thirty-six per cent of well-adjusted mothers as well as 75 per cent of the 'specifically over-reacting' mothers were not completely satisfied with the diagnostic consulation. The main target of dissatisfaction was the physician, not the surgeon or nurse who were thought to 'do something'. While parents may sometimes misinterpret what is said due to anxiety, doctors sometimes are too professionally cautious, or concentrate too much on the physical aspects of cardiac disorder.

57 OFFORD, D.R. and APONTE, J.F. (1967)

'Distortion of disability and effect on family life', *Journal of the American Academy of Child Psychiatry*, 6, 3, 499—511.

Contrary to the expectations of the authors, children who had symptoms from congenital heart disease did not differ from children with congenital heart disease but no symptoms in personal adjustment (as evaluated by a psychiatrist from a battery of psychological tests and an interview); mothers of the children with symptoms were not more over-protective (measured by restrictions not advised by the physician which were placed on the child) nor was the family life of this group more affected by the disorder. The mother's perception of the illness was the key factor in its effect on family life. Mothers who over-estimated the severity of the child's defect (compared with the cardiologist's rating) had the highest over-protection scores, followed by mothers who underestimated the severity, while over-protection was least for those who saw the child's defect accurately; families of the over-estimating mothers were also the most affected by the heart defect and those of mothers with accurate perceptions were least affected. No significant differences were found, though, between child adjustment in the three groups. Mothers who had lived longest with the illness were most likely to over-rate its severity. There was also some tendency for the mother's perception of the severity of the defect to be related to social class — for boys the mother was most likely to distort the severity if the husband had a low occupation level, while for girls distortion was more likely if the occupational level was high — a physical defect being more of an obstacle to the life chances of a boy at the lower socio-economic level and to a girl at the higher level. Subjects were 19 children, aged four to 15 years, admitted to the University of Florida Teaching Hospital for cardiac evaluation, and their mothers.

58 LINDER, R. (1970)

'Mothers of disabled children — the value of weekly group meetings', *Developmental Medicine and Child Neurology*, 12, 202—6.

Group meetings, held over a period of three months, for mothers of children with muscular dystrophy, cerebral palsy and cardiac anomalies are discussed. Meeting others with similar problems helped to overcome the mothers' feelings of isolation.

59 HEFFERMAN, A. (1971)

'An experiment in group therapy with mothers of diabetic children', in R.L. Noland (Ed.) *Counselling parents of the ill and handicapped.* Springfield, Illinois, Charles C. Thomas, pp. 423—31.

Group therapy, over a two-year period, enabled mothers of diabetic children to become more relaxed and confident in their management of the diabetes, gave them increased understanding of their children's reactions to the illness and helped them to handle the children better.

60 MATTSSON, A. and AGLE, D.P. (1972)

'Group therapy with parents of hemophiliacs: therapeutic process and observations of parental adaptation to chronic illness in children', *Journal of the American Academy of Child Psychiatry*, 11, 3, 558—71.

Ten parents of young haemophiliacs took part in a series of 25 weekly group meetings led by a child and a general psychiatrist. At first parents discussed distressing events connected with their children's haemophilia, family hardships, difficulties in achieving appropriate child-rearing methods and parental feelings. After about six weeks group cohesiveness began to emerge and they were able to express negative, hostile and resentful feelings. After about two months parents began to realize that they used many of the same methods to cope with their uncomfortable feelings. Towards the end of the series parents increased in self-esteem and their feelings of isolation diminished. They were able to use more appropriate child-rearing methods, e.g. allowing physical activities with a minimum of supervision. A follow-up after 2 years showed that parents had continued to gain in self-confidence and that their child-rearing methods were generally appropriate.

61 WATSON, A. (1972) 'A study of family attitudes to children with diabetes', *Community Medicine*, 128, 5, 122—5.

In this exploratory study, 15 families randomly selected from all families with diabetic children identified in two London Boroughs, were interviewed in their homes. Initial reactions were shock at the diagnosis (although four parents were relieved it was no worse), followed by anxiety about the technical knowledge needed for diabetic management. Parents felt that they had no opportunity to discuss their feelings about the diagnosis. The emphasis was on management, but teaching of parents at the eight hospitals attended by the children was only barely or less than adequate (except at one hospital with a relatively large child diabetic population). Few parents (five) received home visits from any professional worker in the first few weeks although these would have been welcomed. By the time of the interview 11 families could cope with management techniques. Nevertheless the interviewer considered that eight of the 15 parents had an unacceptably high level of anxiety and stress; distress was related to inadequate understanding of diabetes and lack of confidence in being able to control the child's diabetes, both of which were found mainly in lower social class parents. From interviews with the schools attended by the children it was found that there was little anxiety about having a diabetic pupil but also little knowledge of the illness and its management, although dietary needs were understood. Parents turned to the hospital for advice about diabetes, but hospitals were generally only concerned with the child's medical condition and not his social situation. Communication between the hospitals and the local authorities (at present very rare) suggesting the need for advice and support for some families and between the hospitals and the schools (at present non-existent), to give them initial information, would help to solve some of the problems.

SECTION III   Educational attainments

There is very little research on the educational attainments of children with physical disorders not involving the brain. A recent study has been made, though, which compares the intelligence and educational attainments of all 10-to 12-year-old children with physical disorders living on the Isle of Wight with those of the general population (Yule and Rutter, 1970). The children with physical disorders (excluding those with asthma and exzema) were found, on average, to be slightly below the control group in intelligence. Significantly more of the children with physical disorders (16·67 per cent) than of the general population (5·4 per cent) were reading at a level 28 months or more below that expected for their age and intelligence. At least part of the explanation for this educational retardation was found in the high absence from school rate of the children with physical disorders. Again, of course, these findings do not necessarily apply to all the disorders under review and it is useful to consider the available research for each condition separately.

CARDIAC DISORDERS

There appears to be an almost complete lack of research on the educational attainments of cardiac children. There has been considerable interest, though, in the intelligence of children with congenital heart disease, particularly of those with cyanosis. Children with cyanotic heart defects have lowered blood-oxygen levels and there is a possibility that this may have a damaging effect on intelligence.

Although some research has found no significant difference between the average intelligence of children with congenital heart disease (excluding those having conditions associated with mental retardation) and matched non-handicapped controls (Reed, 1959) other studies have found the cardiac children to be slightly lower in intelligence but within the normal range (Linde et al., 1967; Drash and Money, 1968).

49

In all available studies which examine cyanotic and acyanotic children separately, the cyanotic children have lower average IQs, although still within the normal range (Schlange, 1962; Linde *et al.*, 1967; Rasof *et al.*, 1967; Feldt *et al.*, 1969).

It is not yet clear why cyanotic children have lower intelligence. While it remains possible that the lowered arterial oxygen saturation is the primary factor findings of the study carried out by Linde, Rasof and their associates (Linde *et al.*, 1967; Rasof *et al.*, 1967) suggest that the associated physical incapacity may be of greater importance as it interferes with the child's early manipulative experiences. The relationship found between incapacity and intelligence in young children tended to disappear in older children. The intelligence of the older cyanotic children was significantly higher than that of the younger children. It appears from this study that cyanotic children are able to catch up on experiences after they learn to walk and are also able to perform better on the measures of intelligence used for older groups, which emphasise verbal abilities (Stanford Binet), rather than those used in the early years, which rely mainly on sensory-motor functions (Cattell and Gesell scales).

Findings of a later study, however (Feldt *et al.*, 1969) did not support the view that early environmental deprivation is a major factor in the lowered intelligence of cyanotic children. In this research older cyanotic children did not score higher on intelligence tests than younger children. Feldt and his co-workers, though, found an association between small head circumference, growth failure and low intelligence. Possible explanations put forward by the authors are that an adverse pre-natal factor simultaneously affects the developing heart, brain and other tissues of the developing foetus, or that infant malnutrition, connected with the cardiac defect, results in deficiencies in brain development and growth. Nevertheless it may be that reduced environmental experiences, decreased social contacts and school absences lower the intelligence of older cyanotic children (Linde *et al.*, 1967), and are the main factors responsible in some cases. The causes of the less than average intelligence of children with cyanotic heart disease need further investigation.

In general the IQ of children with congenital heart disease is found to be higher after operation than pre-operatively (Drash and Money, 1968; Landtman *et al.*, 1968; Linde *et al.*, 1970), although it may decrease for some, at least in the immediate post-operative period (Drash and Money, 1968). Linde and his associates found only a small improvement on average in acyanotic children who had undergone surgery (unoperated acyanotic children also improved), but the major change occurred in the cyanotic children who had been operated upon. The change is attributed to their improved physical capacity. Landtman *et al.*, (1968) found an increase of more than ten IQ points in 30 children while only six decreased by this amount. The authors attribute the increase to the improved mother-child relationships found after the operation.

DIABETES

Research on intelligence and educational attainments of diabetic children is meagre in the recent period. While a number of studies since the 1920s have investigated the intelligence of diabetic children most did not take into account socio-economic background, which is known to be related to intelligence, and few considered academic achievements (Ack *et al.*, 1961). Two studies in the 1960s (Ack *et al.*, 1961; Hiltman and Luking, 1966) both found diabetic children to have normal intelligence. Educational attainments of diabetic children also appear to be similar to those of non-handicapped children (Sterky, 1963; Weil and Ack, 1964). Sterky found no significant differences between the school achievements of diabetic school-children in Stockholm and their matched controls. The proportion of diabetic children in special classes was the same as that of non-diabetic children. Weil and Ack found that the reading and arithmetic achievements (California Achievement Tests) of the diabetic children were not significantly different from those expected from their mental ages. Diabetic children performed as well in relation to mental age as their non-diabetic siblings. Nevertheless there are reports that a relatively high proportion of diabetic children have academic difficulties (Etzwiler and Sines, 1962; Weil and Ack, 1964) and these need further investigation.

HAEMOPHILIA

It is only very recently that a detailed study has been made (in Washington, US) of the academic attainments of haemophiliac boys (Olch, 1971b). In this study intelligence of the children was found to be close to that expected in the normal population. Reading and arithmetic attainments of the haemophiliac children were, though, with some exceptions, below those expected for their ability and the gap between ability and attainments widened with increasing age.

Olch considered that the repeated short absences from school of the haemophiliac boys contributed to their low attainments. In her study one third of the boys missed a quarter of each school year. Findings from British studies are similar (Britten *et al.*, 1966; Haemophilia Society, 1969). In Olch's study about half of the boys had received home tutoring during school absences at some time, but a number of the boys thought this had been intellectually unstimulating. In Britain it has sometimes been difficult to arrange home tutoring for haemophiliac children as this is generally reserved for those who are likely to be absent six weeks or more (Britten *et al.*, 1966). Although the situation has improved, 43 per cent of the 17- to 19-year-olds in the Haemophilia Society's survey (1969) who had long absences from school, still never received home tuition.

While attendance at ordinary school, then, presents problems for the haemophiliac boy, schools for the physically handicapped have been found even more unsatisfactory (Britten *et al.*, 1966; Haemophilia Society, 1969; Boon and Roberts, 1970). Complaints by haemophiliacs who attended these schools that progress was too slow are probably justified. A recent study of a school for the physically handicapped indicates that such schools have to cater for many children who are intellectually backward (Segal, 1971).

The solution that has been suggested by some authors (Britten *et al.*, 1966; Haemophilia Society, 1969) is a special boarding school for severely affected haemophiliacs. The school would have a close association with a Haemophilia Centre. As far as is possible the children's education would be continued during bleeding episodes. Such schools have been successfully established in France (Soulier and Josso, 1966). A contrasting view is that of Olch (1971b). She considers that the need is for special measures to make up for missed school-work, rather than for special schools. Home tuition and special help on the child's return to school should always be provided, and use made of modern methods such as programmed material. It certainly seems desirable to try using all means possible to help the child make up for school absences — and to reduce absences to a minimum by ensuring every child receives the best modern treatment available — before resort is made to a special boarding school. An evaluation of school acheivements when such measures are in use would help in deciding the best future educational policy for haemophiliac children.

Abstracts

62 ACK, M., MILLER, I. and WEIL, W.B. Jr. (1961)

'Intelligence of child with diabetes mellitus', *Pediatrics*, 28, 764—70.

Thirty-eight diabetic children, attending the University Hospitals of Cleveland, were found to be similar in intelligence to their non-diabetic siblings; the 13 children who were under five years of age, though, were lower in intelligence than their controls. There was a tendency for episodes of hypoglycaemia and acidosis to be negatively related to intelligence in children under the age of five, but there was no relationship after this age. It is possible that these metabolic disturbances cause mental impairment in a young child but not in an older child. Alternatively, the stress of diabetes on the young child may cause the intellectual loss.

63 SCHLANGE, H.
(1962)

'Die kerperliche and geistige Entwicklung bei Kindern mit angeberenen Herz-und-Gefassmissbildungen'('Physical and mental development of children with cardiovascular congenital defects'), *Beihefte zum Archiv fur Kinderheilkunde*, 47, 1—61.

Weight, height, and early childhood development did not differ very much in children with congenital heart defects from those in non-handicapped children. Speech retardation and speech disabilities were found in about 45 per cent of the children. Congenital defects other than the heart condition were present in some children. About 22 per cent of the children without cyanosis and 32 per cent of those with cyanosis had IQs below 85.

64 WEIL, W.B. Jr. and
ACK, M. (1964)

'School achievement in juvenile diabetes mellitus', *Diabetes*, 13, 3, 303—6.

A further study of the diabetic children found, in a previous investigation (Ack *et al.*, 1961) to be similar in intelligence to their non-diabetic siblings. Reading and arithmetic achievements of the diabetic children were those expected for their mental age. Performance, in relation to mental age, was similar for the diabetic children and their healthy siblings. Age of onset of diabetes was not related to academic achievements.

65 BRITTEN, M.I.,
SPOONER, J.D.,
DORMANDY, K.M.
and BIGGS, R. (1966)

'The haemophilic boy in school', *British Medical Journal*, ii, 224—8.

The authors argue that a special boarding school for haemophiliac children run in close association with a haemophilia treatment centre is the best solution to the educational problems of many severely affected boys. These children need early and adequate treatment for haemorrhages combined with a good and continuous education which will equip them for a non-manual job in adult life. A questionnaire survey of 518 haemophiliac children and young adults (including an unknown number who were only mildly affected) living in England provided evidence of the type of education haemophiliac children were receiving, of difficulties they encountered and on whether there was support for a special boarding school. Of 332 children of school-age, 201 attended ordinary schools and 131 either went to schools for handicapped children or received home tuition. One hundred and nineteen of the 301 children who attended school missed more than a quarter of school-time. Of the 74 young adults known to be severely affected only 13 had attended ordinary schools throughout their school career and 12 of these 13 boys missed more than a quarter of each term. The procedure for obtaining home tuition during school absences is complicated and is normally only set into motion if the doctor considers the child will be away from school for six weeks or more — only nine children in the survey had received temporary home tuition. Parents of children who had attended schools for the physically handicapped felt that the haemophiliac child had been held back by the low intellectual level of many of the children with other disabilities. Two hundred and ninty-two replies in favour of a special boarding school were received from the parents of the haemophiliac children and the young haemophiliac adults who completed questionnaires.

66 HILTMAN, H. and LUKING, J. (1966)

'Die intelligenz bei diabetischen Kindern im Schulalter' ('Intelligence of diabetic children of school age'), *Acta Paedopsychiatrica*, 33, 1, 11—23.

Intelligence test results of 60 diabetic children aged six to 14 in Germany were analysed and compared with those of 44 control children. While not differing from the normal children in overall mean intelligence level there were some significant differences in subtest results, particularly among the boys. Throughout the diabetic group, verbal IQ was significantly higher than performance IQ at all intelligence levels. Lower performance test achievement in diabetics and other physically handicapped children is attributed to restricted motor activity and lower level of physical well-being.

67 SOULIER, J.P. and JOSSO, F. (Eds.) (1966)

Current studies in hemophilia. Proceedings of the 3rd. Congress of the World Federation of Hemophilia, Paris, 1965. Basel, S. Karger, II Medico-Social Session, 2. 'The hemophiliac at school', pp. 162—91.

Five papers, one by an English author and the others by French authors, discuss the medical and psychological problems of the haemophiliac boy at school. A possible solution is the specialized boarding school for haemophiliacs. One paper, by Dr. Favre-Gilly and his associates, describes a school of this type which has been established in France for seven years.

68 LINDE, L.M., RASOF, B. and DUNN, O.J. (1967)

'Mental development in congenital heart disease', *Journal of Pediatrics*, 71, 2, 198—203.

Another account of the research reported in Rasof *et al.*, 1967 (entry 70).

69 PLESS, I.B., RACKHAM, K. and KELLOCK, T.D. (1967)

'Patterns in the admission of handicapped pupils to residential establishments', *Medical Officer*, 118, 135—9.

An examination of the criteria by which children are selected for placement in special residential schools for the 'delicate'. All records available at the time of admission of each child to a boys' school for asthmatics and a hostel for diabetic children of both sexes (one of three in England and Wales), were analysed. Family problems (e.g. parental illness, financial difficulties, family tensions), appeared to be an important reason for admission, occurring in at least a third of both the asthmatic and the diabetic children. A third of the children had previous behaviour problems. Data on other factors likely to have been relevant, such as a worsening of the child's physical condition before admission or interference by the illness in the child's education, were lacking. If, as seems likely from this study, social rather than medical reasons are responsible for selection in many cases, there is need for greater consultation by the Principal School Medical Officer, who makes the final decision, with all who have knowledge of the child and his environment — from the records general practitioners, for example, appear rarely to be consulted.

70 RASOF, B.,
LINDE, L.M. and
DUNN, O.J. (1967)

'Intellectual development in children with congenital heart disease', *Child Development*, 38, 4, 1043—53.

The question of whether intellectual functioning is adversely affected by lowered blood-oxygen levels in children with cyanotic heart disease has been of concern to physicians and parents for a long time. In this study 98 children with cyanotic congenital heart disease were found to score significantly lower in intelligence than three other groups of children — 100 children with congenital heart disease but no cyanosis, 81 healthy siblings of the cardiac children and 40 normal children (Gesell, Cattell and Stanford Binet scales). Children in whom congenital heart disease was part of a syndrome including mental retardation had been excluded from the samples. The average IQ of the cyanotic children was within the normal range at every age level and some had very high scores. Cyanotic children showed developmental delays in walking and speaking phrases compared with the acyanotic and normal children. The differences in intellectual level between the groups could not be accounted for by differences in factors such as age, sex, socio-economic level, or maternal attitudes. In the younger cardiac children (those tested by the Cattell), though, a relationship was found between the level of incapacity and intelligence, but the relationship tended to disappear in the older cardiac children. It is possible that the delay in mental development of the younger children is due to the defect itself — to the lowered arterial oxygen saturation. It is more likely that the associated physical incapacity is the factor of primary importance. The relationship between incapacity and intelligence probably exists in the younger group because tests for this age range rely heavily on sensory-motor functions — and the child's physical incapacity limits both his manipulative experience and his responsiveness and energy in performing the tasks. The relationship tends to disappear in older children both because tests for this group emphasize verbal abilities and because the cardiac child tends to make up on early experience after he begins to walk. (See also Linde *et al.*, 1966 and 1970).

71 BRONKS, I.G. and
BLACKBURN, E.K.
(1968)

'A socio-medical study of haemophilia and related states', *British Journal of Preventive and Social Medicine*, 22, 68—72.

A questionnaire survey carried out in 1964 of 135 patients with haemophilia or related disorders who had been referred to the Department of Haematology at the Sheffield Royal Infirmary in the previous ten years. Forty-four were classified as being mildly affected (excessive haemorrhage after major injuries or operations), 21 as moderately affected (bruising abnormally easily; severe bleeding after minor injury and after surigcal operations), and 70 as severely affected (abnormal bleeding after minor injuries). 57·1 per cent of those aged over 11 years had attended secondary modern schools and 17·1 per cent grammar schools; only 11 attended special schools and only three children did not go to school at all after the age of 11. School-leaving age compared favourably with that of the general population. Seventy-seven per cent of the 87 subjects who had left school were working. Sixty-five per cent of those who were severely affected were employed; only in this group were there any (42·5 per cent) who had been at work for less than 60 per cent of the time in the previous five years. 49·4 per cent of the subjects were married (significantly lower than for the general population) — there were no significant differences between the proportions of those married in the different grades of severity. The percentages of those in employment and married were very similar to those found by Katz (1963). Only four subjects were living alone. Nine subjects (6·7 per cent) stated that they had seen a psychiatrist, although only six had actually received psychiatric treatment. These figures appear to be comparable to those in the general population, suggesting that haemophilia does not cause overt psychiatric illness. Evidence on whether bleeding can be induced by emotional stress was inconclusive.

72 DRASH, P.W. and
MONEY, J. (1968)

'Statural and intellectual growth in congenital heart disease, in growth hormone deficiency and in sibling controls', in D.B. Cheek (Ed.) *Human growth. Body composition, cell growth, energy and intelligence.* Philadelphia, Lea and Febiger, pp. 606—15.

The intelligence distributions of 20 children with unoperated congenital heart disorders and of ten children with congenital heart disorders who had undergone surgery were very close to the expected normal distribution. The mean IQ, though, of the post-operative group was slightly higher than that of the pre-operative group. Two of four children who had undergone open-heart surgery decreased considerably in performance IQ after the operation. The mean IQ of the cardiac group as a whole was 7·59 IQ points lower than that of their normal siblings. The unoperated cardiac children were slightly below average in height and there was a significant degree of correlation between height and intelligence in this group. The low intelligence was as likely to have been the consequence of the general low socio-economic status of this group or an artifact of sampling as to be connected with the growth retardation. No correlation between height and intelligence was found in a group of hypopituitary dwarfs with severe growth retardation.

73 FELDT, R.H., EWERT, J.C., STICKLER, G.B. and WEIDMAN, W.H. (1969)

'Children with congenital heart disease. Motor development and intelligence', *American Journal of Diseases of Children*, 117, 3, 281—7.

An investigation of factors which may be the cause of intellectual retardation in children with congenital heart disease. Subjects were 411 children (aged two to 17 years) with congenital heart defects, seen consecutively at a clinic over a six month period (children with clinically recognizable diseases that may affect mental development, e.g. mongolism, maternal rubella syndrome, were excluded). In 78 children, chosen randomly for psychometric testing (Cattell Infant Scale or Stanford Binet), nine per cent of the acyanotic patients and 44 per cent of the cyanotic patients had IQs below 90. Ten children had a small head circumference (more than two standard deviations below the mean for their age and sex) and all were intellectually retarded. Ten children showed growth failure (height and weight more than two standard deviations below the mean); six of these children were intellectually retarded, four also having a small head circumference. No relationship was found between the severity of the cardiac defect or environmental deprivation (assuming that environmental stimulation increases in older children) and intelligence scores. In the remaining 333 subjects, whose intelligence was evaluated by clinical assessment, a similar relationship was found between intellectual retardation, small head circumference and growth failure. In the study as a whole 31 (14 per cent) of 226 children whose head circumference was measured had a small circumference, a higher incidence than would be expected in the general population, and all but one were intellectually retarded. Small head circumference thus seems to be one factor that may be responsible for intellectual retardation in children with cardiac defects. A high percentage of children in the study who had growth failure also had intellectual retardation and a small head circumference. This could be due to a teratogenic effect on the development of heart, brain and other tissues of the foetus, or, alternatively, infant malnutrition in conjunction with the cardiac defect could result in failure of normal brain development.

74 HAEMOPHILIA SOCIETY (1969)

Survey of adult haemophiliacs. Report on education. London, Haemophilia Society, 15pp.

In a survey of 503 adult haemophiliacs known to the Haemophilia Society over half were found to have lost more than a quarter of their schooling, (the age group with least schooling lost was the youngest, the 17 to 19 age group, but 62 per cent had still lost more than a quarter). The amount of time lost was related to the severity of the condition, 81 per cent of the crippled and 48 per cent of the non-crippled losing more than a quarter of their schooling. The availability of home tuition was found to have increased in recent years, 57 per cent of those in the 17 to 19 years old group, who had long absences, receiving home tuition. Comparing the age groups there was a move away from ordinary to special schooling at both primary and secondary levels but the proportion attending grammar schools increased. Twenty-five per cent of the 17 to 19 years old group had attended a grammar school, 14 per cent a secondary modern school, 28 per cent a special day or boarding school, six per cent a private school and 26 per cent had home tuition. Children who were crippled were somewhat less likely to attend ordinary schools. Of those in the 20 to 24 age group, 19 per cent had been to Technical or Art College, 10 per cent to University or Teachers' Training College and 13 per cent had other training. The survey showed the importance of education for employment success of a haemophiliac — taking into account the proportion crippled, 14 per cent unemployment would have been expected among those who had attended grammar schools while only six per cent were actually found to be unemployed; in contrast, 22·5 per cent unemployment would have been expected among those who did not attend any secondary school, but 39 per cent was found. It is suggested that the best solution to the educational problems of the haemophiliac boy is a special boarding school for haemophiliacs where education can continue, as far as is possible, during bleeding episodes.

75 HONZIK, M.P.,
COLLART, D.S.,
ROBINSON, S.J.
and FINLEY, K.H.
(1969)

'Sex differences in verbal and performance IQs of children undergoing open-heart surgery', *Science*, 164, 3878, 445—7.

In normal samples no significant differences are found between the mental abilities of boys and girls, though girls do tend to be superior on tests of verbal ability while boys are superior on arithmetic tests and tests of spatial reasoning. Sixty boys and 58 girls (aged five to 16 years) were tested approximately six months after open heart surgery on the Wechsler Intelligence Scale for Children. Contrary to the usual findings the girls tended to have significantly poorer scores on the verbal subscale than the boys. For boys the mean verbal IQ (104·2) did not differ significantly from the mean performance IQ (105·2). In contrast, the mean verbal IQ (95·8) of the girls was significantly lower than their mean performance IQ (99·5). When another sample of 22 boys and 18 girls was tested on the Wechsler before surgery results were in the same direction but were not statistically significant, except for a vocabulary subtest where the boys were significantly superior. Comparisons of the pre-operative sample and an enlarged post-operative sample with the normal distribution of IQ showed that the boys' verbal IQ distributions closely approximated the normal curve while the girls' verbal IQ distributions were both clearly below normal. The explanation may be environmental or a sex-associated genetic factor could be the cause.

76 BOON, R.A. and
ROBERTS, D.F.
(1970)

'The social impact of haemophilia', *Journal of Biosocial Science*, 2, 3, 237—64.

A survey of the educational, employment and social problems of 137 haemophiliacs of all ages living in the north of England in 1968. Thirty-eight per cent of the adults and 15 per cent of the children were classified as being mildly affected, 26 per cent of the adults and 10 per cent of the children as moderately affected (partial disability due to haemarthroses) and 14 per cent of the adults and 20 per cent of the children as severely affected (liable to spontaneous bleeds internally or in muscles and joints), the higher proportion of severe cases among the children being due to the earlier diagnosis of the severely affected. Medical advances in treatment should mean that there will be less permanent damage to the joints in the children, but not all parents or general practitioners realized the value of rapid modern treatment. Of the school-age children (45), 29 were or had been attending ordinary primary schools and 14 had gone on to secondary modern schools but none to grammar schools, six attended day schools for the physically handicapped and six were receiving home tuition. Of the 78 adults, 73 had been to ordinary primary schools 63, having gone on to secondary modern schools and six to grammar schools, while six went to schools for the physically handicapped (all were dissatisfied with the standard of education there). About half of the adults but only a few of the children (nine) had lost more than a quarter of their time at school. The limited education of most of the subjects meant that their choice of employment was also limited. Sixty-four of the adults had passed no exams and most started work in unskilled occupations although 20 per cent became apprentices. Fifty per cent had experienced short periods of unemployment and 14 per cent long periods (over a year). Incomes in 1967 were about £5 below the national average of £18.80 (excluding those who earned more than £30 a week). Nevertheless 55 per cent of the adult haemophiliacs were married. It is concluded that co-operation of the medical, education and social services should enable those who are children at present to become integrated into society as useful members.

77 KATZ, A.H. (1970b) *Hemophilia. A study in hope and reality.* Springfield, Illinois, Charles C. Thomas. (Especially, Chapter 6, 'The education of hemophiliacs'; Chapter 7, 'Making a living'; and Chapter 8, 'Some special conditions: hemophilia and work') pp. 39—88.

In a study of 1,055 haemophiliacs over the age of 16 (see also Goldy and Katz, 1963; Katz, 1963 and 1966) it was found that 65 per cent of the sample had been educated at ordinary elementary schools and 14 per cent had received ordinary schooling as well as special schooling or home tuition; 64 per cent were or had been attending high school but 34 per cent did not complete high school; 23 per cent received education beyond high school level, 12 per cent graduating from college. From discussions with haemophiliacs and their families and with school teachers and administrators it appears that the academic achievements of the haemophiliac boy are generally below those expected for age and intelligence. To improve the quality of education for haemophiliacs teachers and administrators need to acquire a greater understanding of haemophilia, so that fears and misconceptions are allayed and the child can be comfortably accepted in an ordinary class; provision of tuition during absences from school, whether in hospital or at home, is also needed. Eighty-two per cent of the haemophiliacs in the survey were currently employed or still at school. There was a far higher rate of unemployment (20 per cent), though, than among the general population (4·6 per cent). Twenty-three per cent were in professional or managerial jobs or owned their own businesses, 18 per cent were labourers and 54 per cent were in white collar or similar occupations. No real relationship was found betweent the severity of the illness and kind of occupation. Income for the employed tended to be higher than in the general population. A comparison was made between the characteristics of the 'unsuccessful' (unemployed seven months or more) (105) and the 'successful' (employed) (447) (see also Katz, 1966). The illness was more often of low severity in the 'successful' (in 50 per cent) than in the 'unsuccessful' (25 per cent). Subjects in the small group (26) who were 'unsuccessful' although their illness was of low severity tended to emphasize their physical disability and to have 'given up', many having left school at an early age. Those who were 'unsuccessful' but whose illness was of high severity had to face real problems, but they probably tended to take a more negative attitude of themselves than did the 'successful'. The 'successful' subjects whose illness was of high severity (70) had tried to de-emphasize their handicap and aimed at living a normal life.

78 RAUBER, N. (1970)

'Enquêts sur la scolarisation des enfants handicapés physiques et malades chroniques en milieu scolaire normal' ('Surveys on physically handicapped and chronically ill children in ordinary schools'), *Revue D'Hygiène et Médicine Scolaires et Universitaires*, 23, 3, 191—205.

A study of 1,310 children with physical handicaps and disorders (75 per cent with motor handicaps, 5·7 per cent cardiac disorders, seven per cent diabetes, 5·5 per cent epilepsy, 5·7 per cent asthma and two per cent haemophilia), 96 per cent of whom were attending ordinary schools. Teachers felt that 80 to 87 per cent of the children were correctly placed in ordinary schools. Eighty to 90 per cent were thought to be well-integrated. Absence from school was a problem in most of the handicapping conditions.

79 YULE, W. and RUTTER, M. (1970)

'Educational aspects of physical disorder', in M. Rutter, J. Tizard and K. Whitmore (Eds.) *Education, health and behaviour*. London, Longman, pp. 297—308.

The intelligence of 10 to 12-year-old children with physical disorders not involving the brain (orthopaedic disabilities, heart disease, diabetes mainly — asthma and eczema excluded) living in the Isle of Wight was found to be slightly lower than that of the general population (shortened version of the Wechsler Intelligence Scale for Children). 16·67 per cent of these children were reading at a level at least 28 months below that expected for their age and intelligence, compared with 5·4 per cent in the control group (Neale Analysis of Reading Ability). An important factor in this backwardness appears to be absence from school. Fifteen of the 16 children who were 28 months retarded in reading had been absent from school 70·9 half days in the previous school-year, compared with 48·1 for the rest of the children with physical disorders. Absence from school probably also accounts for the slightly lowered intelligence of these children. The loss of confidence which may result from repeated short absences from school was probably as important a factor in the educational retardation of these children as the actual school work missed.

80 OLCH, D. (1971b)

'Effects of hemophilia upon intellectual growth and academic achievement', *Journal of Genetic Psychology*, 119, 63—74.

A study of the intellectual and educational functioning of 45 haemophiliac boys and young men, aged two to 21 years, who were on the files of a major treatment centre in the United States. There was an absence of subjects from the lowest socio-economic level. Intelligence tended to be in the high average range (average IQ 109·3 — Stanford Binet and Wechsler intelligence scales). Intellectual strengths and weaknesses tended to be related to the children's experiences — they were strong in areas involving manipulation of objects or needing factual knowledge, probably due to the time spent making models, reading and watching television when recovering from bleeding episodes but they were relatively weak in areas needing some understanding of social situations. Academic achievements were generally below the children's level of ability; one-third read below grade level and two-thirds were below grade level in arithmetic. With increasing age the academic achievements of the haemophiliac child declined in relation to their potential ability. On average the haemophiliac boys missed twice as much schooling as the general school population; often home tutoring was not given as the individual school absences were brief and, on the whole, little special help was provided on the child's return to school. School absences, though, were not clearly related to academic achievements; the main determinants of achievement were intelligence and socio-economic level, certain personality characteristics also playing a part. The author concludes that the haemophiliac child should be given special consideration rather than special schooling. There should be provisions for making up missed school-work, even when absences are short.

81 SEGAL, S.S. (1971)   *From care to education.* William Heinemann Medical Books, 202pp.

A survey of one special school for the physically handicapped, with the primary purpose of investigating the nature and extent of educational backwardness. In the three school years from 1966—8 the five main handicaps, accounting for over 65 per cent of the school's population, were cerebral palsy (30 to 40 per cent), poliomyelitis (nine to 11 per cent), spina bifida (five to ten per cent), heart conditions (eight to 11 per cent) and muscular dystrophy (four to eight per cent), a similar pattern to that found nationally. In July 1967 when a series of five standardized tests was given to all pupils over the age of seven years, backwardness was found in basic subjects in 65 to 89 per cent of children both at the primary and secondary level. Intelligence tests made on four age-groups of pupils showed that the school population was below average in intellectual ability, 65 per cent having IQs of 85 or below. The largest number of intellectually backward children was in the cerebral palsy group, 85·6 per cent having IQs below 85, while the figure for those with heart conditions was 58·3 per cent. 61·8 per cent of the pupils were in the maladjusted/unsettled categories of the Bristol Social Adjustment Guide. The proportions of emotional disorder were not significantly different among the brain damaged group and the group without brain damage. Although there was some relationship between emotional disorder and educational backwardness, between 40 and 71 per cent in the emotionally stable/quasi-stable group were also backward on one of the attainment tests. It is concluded that the school cannot aim at a normal pattern of education without doing a disservice to the majority of the pupils.

82 DEPARTMENT OF EDUCATION AND SCIENCE (1972a)

'Schools for delicate children', *in Aspects of special education,* Education Survey 17. London, HMSO, pp. 2—21.

A survey by HM Inspectors during 1970—1 of all 52 schools (20 day, 30 residential, two mixed) which cater for 'delicate' children. Of the 4,443 pupils, 1,512 had asthma and 641 other respiratory disorders. Several schools reported that there was an increase in the number of children with more serious physical disorders such as congenital heart disease, 'brittle bones', diabetes and haemophilia — the number of pupils classified as having disorders of the cardio-vascular system was 95, and 55 had diabetes. About a quarter of the children had emotional or behaviour problems — this being the primary reason for admittance in many cases. Twenty per cent of the children had adverse social circumstances at home. Three hundred and fourteen were intellectually retarded, and a majority of all the pupils were educationally retarded. Turnover was considerable, many pupils leaving at 11 and transferring to an ordinary secondary school. The varying time spent at the school and the wide range of ability presented many educational difficulties. Nevertheless the majority of schools were providing stimulating learning situations at the primary level. Problems were greater at the secondary level. One solution was to arrange for the older pupils to join other schools in the area for some lessons; 16 schools had such arrangements. Thirty schools managed to enter some pupils for external examinations. Most of the schools were small and they provided a warm and encouraging atmosphere — in some cases, though, they were also too undemanding, the pupils being overdependent as a result. More supporting services, particularly visits from an educational psychologist to advise on the many learning problems, and access to psychiatric help, are needed.

SECTION IV General

Articles summarized in this section are mainly concerned with the treatment and management of children with cardiac conditions, diabetes and haemophilia. Some give factual information about the conditions. Psychological problems of the child and his family, educational and employment problems are discussed by a number of authors.

Abstracts

83 COOPER, H. (1959)

'Psychological aspects of congenital heart disease', *South African Medical Journal*, 33, 17, 349—52.

A cardiac clinic should provide psychological assistance for both the child with a congenital heart defect and his parents during the pre-operative years. Psychological problems may arise from the child's difficulty in accomplishing physical activities and the consequent inability to keep up with peers or they may stem from faulty parental attitudes produced by feelings of guilt or pathological anxiety. Psychological handling of the child at the actual time of surgery is also discussed.

84 KATZ, A.H. (1959)

'Some psychosocial problems in hemophilia', *Social Casework*, 40, 321—6.

The medical problems of haemophilia and the resulting psychological, practical and financial (in the United States) problems for the family are described. Counselling for both the child and the parents is essential — early vocational counselling is particularly important as the haemophiliac adolescent and young adult without a suitable occupation is liable to become dependent and apathetic.

85 ONGLEY, P.A. and DuSHANE, J.W. (1961)

'Rehabilitation of the child with congenital heart disease', *American Journal of Cardiology*, 7, 335—9.

Treatment and management are discussed for cardiac children: (a) with surgically correctable heart defects; (b) with defects which can be only partially corrected by surgery or who have post-operative heart block; (c) who can be helped medically but not surgically; (d) for whom no satisfactory treatment is available at present. General medical management, physical activity and the social and emotional adjustment of the child are considered.

86 BELMONTE, M.M. (1963)

'The future of the diabetic child', *Canadian Medical Association Journal*, 88, 22, 1112—6.

Research is reviewed on the relationship between the vascular complications of diabetes and control, on diet and on the use of oral hypoglycaemic agents.

87 GEIST, H. (1964)

The psychological aspects of diabetes. Springfield, Illinois, Charles C. Thomas, 81pp.

One section of this book describes the psychological problems that may be caused by juvenile diabetes and its management and discusses the best ways of dealing with them — dietary restrictions, stigma of diabetes, regulation of daily activities, parental reactions and the physiological and psychological changes of adolescence may all give rise to problems. Other aspects covered include: a review of the role of psychological factors in the causation of diabetes and of the effect of stress on the course of the illness; discussion of the causes and control of diabetes.

88 INGRAM, G.I.C. (1965)

'Some problems of social management in haemophilia', *British Journal of Clinical Practice*, 19, 9, 495—9.

Suggestions are made for meeting some of the problems of haemophilia that arise during infancy, school-age and adult life. At the primary school stage it may be helpful to tell teachers in advance something about haemophilia, to reassure them that the child will not bleed to death from minor injuries and warn that he may have to be absent from school periodically. Local education authorities should be approached about home tuition during school absences, and asked if the usual requirement that the child is likely to be away from school for at least a month can be waived. At secondary level the boy should attend an ordinary school if possible and a preliminary interview with the prospective headmaster to give him all necessary information should be arranged. By this age the boy's response to minor injury should be known and he should take the maximum part possible in sports compatible with this. Once the haemophiliac is old enough to understand his own limitations he should be restricted as little as possible — over-protection may be more harmful than a certain amount of accidental injury.

89 BIGGS, R. and MacFARLANE, R.G. (Eds.) (1966)

Treatment of haemophilia and other coagulation disorders. Oxford, Blackwell, 391pp (Especially Chapters IV and XVII).

Written by specialists, chapters in this book discuss many aspects of the treatment of the haemophiliac patient. Chapters IV and XVII include advice on management of the child at home.

90 HAEMOPHILIA SOCIETY (1966)

Survey of adult haemophiliacs. Preliminary report. London, Haemophilia Society, 11pp.

First report of a survey of 503 adult haemophiliacs living in the United Kingdom. Aspects covered include personal characteristics of the haemophiliacs, social life, availability of treatment, financial and employment problems. It is concluded that haemophiliacs aim to achieve normality in their lives and succeed to a remarkable degree despite inadequacies in treatment and education and misunderstanding of the condition by the general public and even some of the medical profession. (See also Haemophilia Society, 1969).

91 HAY, J.D. (1966)

'Care of children with chronic heart disease', in *Child Care.* London, British Medical Association, pp.279—86.

The main responsibilities of the family doctor are: (1) explanation to the parents — and child himself, if he is old enough — of the nature of the heart condition; (2) supervision of the child's care at home and school; (3) prompt treatment of infections. The maximum activity compatible with the child's cardiac capacity should be encouraged — this promotes both good general health and emotional adjustment.

92 AGLE, D.P. and MATTSSON, A. (1968)

'Psychiatric and social care of patients with hereditary hemorrhagic disease', *Modern Treatment*, 5,1,111—24.

For successful treatment of the haemophiliac patient the physician must both be aware of the emotional stresses that affect the child and his family and be able to promote those activities which lead to the most satisfactory adjustment. Aspects discussed by the authors include: the impact of haemophilia on the child and his parents; psychiatric syndromes that may occur in haemophiliacs; realistic responses to the illness; parental attitudes; necessity of encouraging judgement and self-reliance in the haemophiliac child; the question of what constitutes a reasonable level of physical activity; psychological management of bleeding episodes; problems of rebellion in adolescence; vocational choice.

93 BOSSINA, K.K. (1968)

'Social aspects of paediatric cardiology — the child with heart disease in the community', in H. Watson (Ed.) *Paediatric Cardiology.* London, Lloyd-Luke (Medical Books), pp.946—50.

Implications of a diagnosis of congenital heart disease for the child and his family are discussed. Fear of the illness, disappointment, annoyance, and feeling different from others may lead to neurosis in the child. Over-protection by parents will only worsen matters — the child should be treated as much like his normal siblings as possible. Special restrictions in sport are seldom necessary as children who need to restrict their activities usually do this themselves — unnecessary restrictions not only lead to the child being isolated from his peers but also result in poor muscle tone, easy fatigue and inadequate motor co-ordination. The article ends with advice on the preventive medical management of the child with heart disease.

94 WEIL, W.B. Jr. (1968)

'Current concepts: juvenile diabetes mellitus', *New England Journal of Medicine,* 278, 15, 829—31.

Many problems in diabetes are unresolved and are the subjects of current discussion, including: the relationship between control and late complications in the illness; aetiology; the course of the illness; prescribed or self-selected diet; assessment of control; the age at which the diabetic child should assume responsibility for his own management; the purpose and value of summer camps.

95 CHEST AND HEART ASSOCIATION (1969)

Congenital heart disease. Leaflet H. 155. London, Chest and Heart Association, 10pp.

Information for parents about congenital heart defects. Advice on how to prepare the child for diagnostic tests or operation is also given.

96 COLLINS, J. (1969)

'Haemophilia — a social worker's view', *Medical Social Work,* 22, 4, 111—17.

This article gives some factual information on haemophilia and its treatment. Problems of schooling, employment and marriage are also briefly discussed. The author's views are based on her experience as a medical social worker at the Cardiff Royal Infirmary Medical Unit.

97 KATZ, A.H. (1970c)

Hemophilia. A study in hope and reality. Springfield, Illinois, Charles C. Thomas, 159pp.

An examination of the social and psychological problems of haemophilia. Based on his own study of 1055 adult haemophiliacs living in the United States and on the research findings of others the author describes the personal and social characteristics of haemophiliacs and discusses family, educational and employment problems. One chapter is concerned with haemophiliacs' views of themselves and their situation. (See also Katz, 1970a and b).

98 NEILL, C.A. (1970)

'The cardiac child and his family', in M. Debuskey (Ed.) *The chronically ill child and his family.* Springfield, Illinois, Charles C. Thomas, pp.33—51.

Problems faced by the parents during the infancy of a child with a cardiac defect, and problems of the child himself and his family during the school-years and adolescence are discussed.

99 RIZZA, C.R. (1970)

'The management of haemophilia', *Practitioner*, 204, 763—72.
Management and treatment of the haemophiliac patient are discussed. Full use of the specialised haemophilia centres that have been set up throughout the United Kingdom is necessary if the patient is to receive the best treatment. Close collaboration is needed between the general practitioner, hospital, teachers and social workers to ensure that the boy grows up to lead as normal a life as possible with the minimum of crippling. Parents should be given some guide lines by which to judge if bleeds need immediate hospital treatment and they should be encouraged to make plans for the child's education at an early stage.

100 YOUNGHUSBAND, E., BIRCHALL, D., DAVIE, R. and KELLMER PRINGLE, M.L. (Eds.) (1970)

Living with handicap. London, National Bureau for Co-operation in Child Care (now National Children's Bureau), 372pp.
The report of a working party of experts set up under the auspices of the National Children's Bureau to review the needs of handicapped children and the adequacy of the existing services for them. Evidence and information was obtained from professional and voluntary organizations, local authorities and from parents of handicapped children. On the basis of these contributions and their own experiences in various disciplines concerned with handicapped children the working party made detailed recommendations on every aspect of their subject.

101 RIZZA, C.R. and BIGGS, R. (1971)

'Haemophilia today', *British Journal of Hospital Medicine*, 6, 3, 343—56.
This article deals mainly with the treatment of bleeding episodes in haemophilia. It is emphasized that management of the patient must be concerned with all the problems he encounters because of the haemophilia and must not solely concentrate on medical treatment.

102 BRITISH DIABETIC ASSOCIATION (1972a)

Childhood and adolescence. Leaflet DH.126. London, British Diabetic Association, 8pp.
Basic information for parents on diabetes and its treatment.

103 BRITISH DIABETIC ASSOCIATION (1972b)

The diabetic at school. Leaflet DH.127. London, British Diabetic Association, 4pp.
Information about diabetes for teachers.

104 COURT, J.M. (1972)

Your child has diabetes. A guide to parents and to their children who have diabetes. Sydney, Ure Smith, 256pp.
Part I explains the condition and its treatment simply, with illustrations. Part II gives detailed information on management — injections, diet, exercise, insulin reactions (hypoglycaemia), urine tests.

One chapter consists of accounts, written by diabetic children, on how they feel about the illness. Part III answers many of the questions the author, a doctor at a Melbourne diabetic clinic, has been asked by diabetic children and their parents. Appendices contain detailed information on diet.

105 DEPARTMENT OF EDUCATION AND SCIENCE (1972b)

'The diabetic child', in *The health of the school child, 1969—70*. HMSO, pp.64—8.

Discussion of the nature, treatment, prevalence and prognosis of childhood diabetes.

106 WORLD HEALTH ORGANIZATION (1972)

Inherited blood clotting disorders. Technical Report Series no.504. Geneva, WHO, 48pp.

Report of a WHO Scientific Group. Recent developments in understanding of the blood clotting disorders and their genetic basis are reviewed. Other aspects covered are: treatment and management of patients, family and social problems, the detection of carriers, genetic counselling and preventive measures.

107 WORLD HEALTH ORGANIZATION, REGIONAL OFFICE FOR EUROPE (1972)

Congenital heart diseases in Europe. Report on a Working Group, Copenhagen, September, 1971. 39pp. (Limited number of copies only available for persons officially or professionally concerned with the field of study from the WHO Regional Office for Europe, Copenhagen).

The report of the working group discusses: aetiology, prevalence and prognosis of congenital heart disease; diagnostic techniques and the need for early detection; management, including medical and surgical treatment and the psychological aspects; organization of services for treatment of patients with congenital heart defects.

Author Index

Numbers refer to bibliographic entry numbers, not pages

Neill, C.A. (1970) 98
Neuhaus, E.C. (1958) 1
Offord, D.R. and Aponte, J.F.
(1967) 57
Olch, D. (1971a) 46, (1971b) 80
Ongley, P.A. and DuShane, J.W.
(1961) 85
Pless, I.B., Rackham, K. and Kellock,
T.D. (1967) 69
Rasof, B., Linde, L.M. and Dunn,
O.J. (1967) 70
Rauber, N. (1970) 78
Reed, M.K. (1959) 2
Richardson, S.A., Hastorf, A.H. and
Dornbusch, S.M. (1964) 18
Rizza, C.R. (1970) 99
Rizza, C.R. and Biggs, R. (1971)
101
Schiff, L.J. (1964) 19
Schlange, H. (1962) 63
Segal, S.S. (1971) 81
Soulier, J.P. and Josso, F. (Eds.)
(1966) 67
Spencer, R.F. and Behar, L. (1969)
35
Stearns, S. (1959) 3

Stein, S.P. and Charles, E. (1971)
47
Sterky, G. (1963) 16
Swift, C.R. and Seidman, F.L. (1964)
20
Swift, C.R., Seidman, F.L. and Stein,
H. (1967) 27
Tietz, W. and Vidmar, J.T. (1972)
49
Treuting, T.F. (1962) 12
Watson, A. (1972) 61
Weil, W.B. Jr. (1968) 94
Weil, W.B. Jr. and Ack, M. (1964)
64
Weil, W.B. Jr. and Sussman, M.B.
(1961) 7, (1967) 28
World Health Organization (1972)
106
World Health Organization, Regional
Office for Europe (1972) 107
Younghusband, E., Birchall, D.,
Davie, R. and Kellmer Pringle,
M.L. (Eds.) (1970) 100
Yule, W. and Rutter, M. (1970)
79